Praise for *Also Human*

'All agree there is a crisis in health care, but this book looks behind the headlines and tots up the human cost of a flawed system. Written with perceptive sympathy for the wounded healer, it is necessary reading for both doctors and patients.'

Hilary Mantel

'Fascinating, troubling, educative. Read Elton and weep and then think, argue and implement what needs doing to support not squander our medics.'

Susie Orbach

'With a compassionate eye for detail and a deep understanding of just how the systems we train and practice in as doctors can fail us as human beings, Caroline Elton offers a crucial and timely reminder that doctors are *Also Human*.'

Atul Gawande, author of *Being Mortal*

'Caroline Elton is an occupational psychologist who has worked with medics for more than 20 years. She is uniquely qualified to comment ... I'd be surprised if anyone who reads it will ever look at doctors in the same light again.'

Guardian

'*Also Human* describes, through a series of case histories... the emotional and psychological problems that doctors can face ... At the heart of this book is the problem of how emotional resilience can be identified in prospective doctors and strengthened in practising doctors. We are fallible human beings, not omniscient gods.'

Henry Marsh, *Sunday Times*

'Doctors are people, too. They possess the same virtues, faults, fears and desires of the rest of us but it's easy for patients to forget this obvious truth. Caroline Elton's revelatory, sometimes disturbing, book, is a welcome reminder of this. For doctors and patients alike, this book is required reading.'

Daily Mail

'Timely, passionately argued.'

British Journal of General Practice

'Her descriptions of the psychological forces underlying the way doctors act ... is fascinating, with succinct explorations.'

Literary Review

'An important, necessary book. *Also Human* shows that doctors are indeed all so human.'

Dean Burnett, author of *The Idiot Brain*

'A shocking indictment of a system of training and supervision that ought to have gone out of fashion and use decades ago. Caroline Elton's incisive prose, and her impatience with the way people display prejudice and poor practice in front of her makes for very good, if highly disturbing, reading. I was horrified by this book, but so glad she has written it.'

Julia Neuberger

'Have you ever wondered what your doctor thinks and feels once you walk out the door? *Also Human* is the uncensored answer – and it's haunting, beautiful, and urgent for all of us to know.'

Johann Hari, author of *Chasing the Scream*

'A vivid, compelling account of how wounded healers may struggle to find healing. Elton has helped hundreds of doctors through crises in their personal and professional lives, and her stories read as an urgent manifesto to reform the caring professions – that they might begin to care for their own. With reference from the psychological literature, as well as her own extensive clinical experience, she examines why some doctors are overwhelmed by the pressures of medicine, while others may even thrive under them.'

Gavin Francis, author of *Shapeshifters: On Medicine & Human Change*

'Shocking … a graphic exposé of the exhaustion, depression, and stress among doctors and it has sent shock waves across the health services.'

Irish Examiner

Also Human

The Inner Lives of Doctors

Caroline Elton

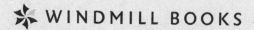

7 9 10 8 6

Windmill Books
20 Vauxhall Bridge Road,
London SW1V 2SA

Windmill Books is part of the Penguin Random House group
of companies whose addresses can be found
at global.penguinrandomhouse.com.

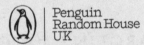

Penguin
Random House
UK

First published by William Heinemann in 2018
First published in paperback by Windmill Books in 2019

www.penguin.co.uk

A CIP catalogue record for this book is available from the British Library.

ISBN 9780099510796

Typeset in 12.5/17 pt Fourniern MT Std
by Integra Software Services Pvt. Ltd, Pondhicherry

Printed and bound in Great Britain by Clays Ltd, Elcograf S.p.A.

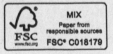

For my family

Mary W is a psychologist who lives in Michigan . . . More than a decade ago, when I was trying to decide whether to go to medical school to become a psychiatrist, I called her to talk about her practice . . . Mary shares my love for northern Michigan and its lakes. Without thinking, she reached for that shared territory for a metaphor.

'The patients we work with have fallen through the ice in the middle of a frozen lake . . . My job – your job should you take this path – is to go out to them, to be with them on the thin ice, and to work with them to get them out of the frigid water. . . . But you must know that if you go out to them on the thin ice, there's a real danger that you'll fall in too. So if you go into this work, you've got to be anchored to the shore. You can reach out one hand to the person in the water,' she cautioned, 'but your other hand needs to have a firm grip on the people and things that connect you to the shore. If you don't, you lose your patients, and you lose yourself.'

Falling into the Fire: A Psychiatrist's Encounters with the Mind in Crisis, Christine Montross

CONTENTS

AUTHOR'S NOTE

A note on client confidentiality which I have taken very seriously. I have changed names and all identifying particulars so as to preserve my clients' anonymity. Before using any personal information in the book (even under the guise of anonymity), I showed each client the draft, invited comment and sought their permission: all were willing to share their experience. Most were willing to do so on the basis that it is this book's aim to help doctors facing career struggles and highlight the extraordinarily difficult pressures that many doctors face.

INTRODUCTION

Medicine in the Mirror

———————————

As the aeroplane wheels touched down on the tarmac I instinctively reached for my mobile phone, like many others around me. The flight from London to Washington DC was only eight hours, so there wasn't much to work through. And there was nothing that a breezy 'out of office' message wouldn't hold at bay for the next eight days. Nothing of concern – until I reached the last email:

Dear Caroline

I have questioned from day one whether medical school was right for me, and since then things have only gotten worse: I have got more depressed and felt more hopeless as I have gone through – persisting always with the hope that things might get better (and everyone around me encouraging me to do so). But I just can't cope with the pressure and stress of hospitals, and the thought of starting work as a doctor fills me with dread.

I am now a month away from finals and very distressed about what to do. I keep trying to tell myself that I just need to pass my finals then can always stop and do something else with my medical degree. But I have no real clue about what I would do instead – and am just as scared that I may regret it if I stop . . .

I am just not sure I will survive working as a doctor, and I'm worried I would get so stressed, anxious and depressed that I would end up either hurting someone else by accident or more likely drive myself to the edge. I am sorry if this comes across quite melodramatic. I really have reached crisis point though and am in desperate need for some sane input.

Leo

I froze. This was not an email to ignore. But how could I provide 'sane input' when I was on the wrong side of the Atlantic? In the taxi to my son's house, I phoned a colleague in order to pass the baton to her – but I only got her answerphone. There was no option but to answer Leo's email myself.

*

Everybody goes to the doctor from time to time. For some, visits are a frequent occurrence, whilst for others they are mercifully rare. But however often we seek medical advice, or need treatment, most of us, quite naturally, tend to be preoccupied with our own concerns, and to make all sorts of assumptions about the doctor who is listening to us, taking our medical history, or cutting into us during an operation. If we think of them at all.

We take it on trust that the doctor is up to the task, and doesn't feel tired or overwhelmed. We rarely consider whether the doctor, like Leo, is terrified of accidentally hurting us. We simply assume that if they are relatively junior, there will be a senior clinician somewhere nearby to answer their questions and ensure that they're doing their job correctly. We tend not to worry whether or not they are bright enough for the job – after all, they will have trained for years and will have passed countless exams to get through medical school and beyond. And when parts of our body are being examined, we don't want to entertain the possibility that doctors may find some patients attractive. We don't wonder if the doctor likes patients at all, finds them disgusting, or resents the responsibility inherent in patient care. Instead we imagine that doctors enjoy their work and find it satisfying to treat patients like us.

For many of us, much of what we know about the medical profession comes from watching television. But neither the medical soap operas, nor the fly-on-the-wall documentaries paint an accurate picture. We don't see junior doctors feeling so overwhelmed by work that they run away in fear. Neither, for ethical reasons, would we be shown doctors telling parents that their baby has died. Yet that's just one of the many traumatic tasks that might be on a doctor's 'to do' list alongside calming down a delusional patient or deciding whether to call a halt on a failing resuscitation attempt. And television, compelling though it may be, is restricted to sights and sounds; it can't convey the smell of decaying flesh, or as one doctor described it to me 'the feel of burnt, crispy, human skin'.

A lot of what doctors do is shielded in secrecy. 'We cannot speak of these things to people outside medicine, because it is too traumatic, too graphic, too much,' wrote one doctor recently, in the *New York Times*. But the writer then flagged up the difficulty of gaining solace through talking to colleagues, as medical culture regards these difficult tasks as 'just the job we do, hardly worth commenting on'. A conspiracy of silence.

This book breaks the silence. Over the last twenty years, working as an occupational psychologist in two unusual roles, I have seen and heard things that are hidden from patients.

I found the first of these roles by chance; while idly flicking through the jobs section of the newspaper I spotted a vacancy on a project that aimed to make hospital consultants more effective teachers. Rather than removing doctors from their clinical duties and sending them en masse to the education department for training, faculty from the education depart-ment went into hospital to shadow the clinicians as they taught their students and junior doctors. Ward rounds, oper-ations or outpatient clinics could continue as normal as clini-cians were observed as they went about their everyday duties. What's more, the educational feedback was more precise: tailored to the specific context in which each particular clini-cian worked.

I applied for the role, and ended up working on the project for the next decade. During this time I shadowed hundreds of consultants; I watched as babies were born, patients were given terminal diagnoses or took their last breaths. My job was to help these consultants become more effective teachers in the different settings across the hospital; in the process I witnessed many extraordinary things.

Alongside this hospital-based role, I also had a more typical job for an occupational psychologist: working as a careers counsellor, helping people sort out the difficulties that they were experiencing in the workplace. For many years my two jobs were separate: some days I observed doctors whilst on others I counselled people in all occupations *other* than medicine. Then in 2006 my two jobs merged. Postgraduate training of doctors in the UK was completely overhauled, junior doctors had to make specialty choice decisions at an earlier point in their careers, and the NHS woke up and realised that there was a need to establish careers support services for doctors.*

In 2008 I was employed by the NHS to set up and run the Careers Unit – a service for all trainee doctors in the seventy-plus hospitals across the capital. Although I hadn't embarked on the observation work to prepare me for this new role, serendipitously the ten years I spent shadowing clinicians turned out to be invaluable. I had seen, for example, anaesthetists or gastro-enterologists or cardiac surgeons in action, so I had a more nuanced understanding of the pleasures and challenges of each specialty than I could ever have acquired from a book.

---

* In this book I focus on the inner lives of doctors. This is not because the other professionals working in healthcare don't matter; they do. They are essential. Instead, the reason is that in both of the roles I have held over the past twenty years, I was solely responsible for supporting doctors and had minimal contact with staff from other professions. I don't want to presume that I have much understanding of the challenges that other professional groups face which is why I have remained silent on the matter.

But the junior doctors who came banging on my door at the Careers Unit didn't only want to talk about choosing the right specialty.* Other themes recurred again and again: coping with the transition from medical school; questioning whether they were suited to the practice of medicine; the impact of exposure to patient suffering; the seeming impossibility of reconciling family and professional demands; the emotional complexity of leaving or abandoning a medical career. These are some of the issues that I explore in this book.

As a psychologist, I saw how medical training often fails to acknowledge that doctors are people too, with their own thoughts, feelings, fantasies and desires. Their training moves them around the country, and separates them from family and friends. They can get ill, or divorced, or fail to find a partner. Some struggle to progress their careers after taking time out to care for their children or elderly parents, others struggle with passing specialty exams. The sexism or racism found in other professional spheres hasn't been surgically excised from medical work. Some doctors feel that they have ended up in the wrong specialty. All of this takes a toll.

All of this needs to be told.

*

It might be tempting to think that the doctors who came to see me were rare outliers – far removed from a notional 'average'

* The remit of the service I set up in 2008 was to support junior doctors; those who had completed their training were sadly not eligible for help. It's for this reason that most of the stories in this book focus on younger doctors – who after all, are the future members of the profession. Alongside my NHS work, I also maintained a small private practice and saw doctors who were not eligible to access free support from the Careers Unit. The stories in the book about consultants or GPs come from the doctors who came to see me privately. Irrespective of where I saw them, all doctors in the book have given me permission to tell their stories.

member of the profession. But this would be false. I am certainly not suggesting that *all* doctors encounter the difficulties described in this book; just as patients don't tend to go the doctor when they are well; doctors don't tend to seek out a psychologist who specialises in career difficulties when they are loving their work. Yet the volume of individuals who came to see me (and continue to do so) indicates that these challenges are far from uncommon.

Moving beyond my own experience, there are numerous studies and editorials published in medical journals that paint a worrying picture of doctors' wellbeing. A tragic example would be the impassioned opinion piece in 2016 written by the Dean of a medical school in New York, where one of the students had recently committed suicide by jumping out of a high window. Referring to research from the Mayo Clinic, he described 'a national epidemic of burnout, depression and suicide amongst medical students'. And he went on to say that the 'root causes' of this epidemic stemmed from

A culture of performance and achievement that for most of our students begins in middle school and relentlessly intensifies for the remainder of their adult lives. Every time students achieve what looks to the rest of us like a successful milestone – getting into a great college, the medical school of their choice, a residency into a competitive clinical specialty – it is to some of them the opening of another door to a haunted house, behind which lie demons, suffocating uncertainty and unimaginable challenges.

A few months before the New York medical student committed suicide, Rose Polge, a junior doctor in the UK, walked into the sea and drowned. This tragedy received widespread newspaper coverage – at least in part because it occurred when junior doctors had taken the unprecedented step of going on strike – the first in forty years – in protest against the imposition of a new working contract.

'Long hours, work-related anxiety and despair at her future in medicine were definite contributors to this awful and final decision,' wrote Rose's parents on the web page of a charity set up to raise money in her memory.

Except it isn't final. The following year another junior doctor disappeared. As with Rose, her car was found abandoned by the sea. What happened next is not known.

Rose's parents were not alone in pointing the finger at the working conditions doctors face in the UK. A 2016 study published in *The Lancet* concluded that GPs' clinical workload was reaching 'saturation point'. Similarly, the quarterly monitoring report from the King's Fund published at the beginning of 2017 noted sustained increases in patient demand, particularly from elderly patients with complex health needs, rising delays in transferring patients out of hospital into social care and severe financial pressures leading to cuts in staffing. These findings were echoed in a survey of nearly 500 junior doctors conducted by the Royal College of Physicians which reported that:

70% worked on a rota that was permanently under-staffed. At least four times per month doctors completed a full day or night shift without having time to eat.

18% had to carry out clinical tasks for which they had not been adequately trained

80% felt their work sometimes or often caused them excessive stress

25% felt their work had a serious impact on their mental health.

But ultimately it's not just doctors who are suffering. It's all of us. The Royal College of Physicians' survey found that nearly a half of doctors felt that poor morale had a serious, or extremely serious, impact on patient safety. Similarly the 2016 General Medical Council survey of junior doctors reported that one in five emergency medicine trainees were concerned about the impact of their workload on patient safety. And another study carried out by researchers at Harvard Medical School reported that paediatric trainees who were suffering from depression made six times more medication errors than their non-depressed colleagues. These researchers also found that the rate of depression amongst these trainees was twice that expected in the general population. Despite these high rates of mental distress, nearly half of the depressed trainees seemed unaware that they were unwell and only a small number were receiving treatment.

*

It's extremely rare for a psychologist to gain such intimate exposure to the day-to-day reality of medical work. In many ways I have been granted an insider's vantage point on the profession. Yet crucially, in both of my roles I was working as an outsider, as a psychologist rather than as a medic. I haven't been socialised into the world of medicine through a long and arduous training process, so things that medical colleagues might take for granted, I have questioned. My training has also given me a psychological lens to interpret what I have seen or been told; I'm often interested in the unconscious reasons that lie beneath some of the decisions doctors make.

But the significance of being a psychologist rather than a doctor goes further. I suspect it's a bit easier for doctors to admit to me that they are struggling at work, than to have the same conversation with another doctor. When their jobs are making them unhappy, doctors often imagine that they are the only ones who feel as they do, and they are wary of voicing their concerns to the senior clinicians who supervise them. And stigma – particularly around mental health issues – is still a very real problem in the medical profession.

There are, of course, a number of books written by exceptional physicians, which provide readers with an extraordinary glimpse into the world of medicine. I have read many of them, and they have enormously enriched my understanding of the profession. But this book is different; it's not describing the personal experience of one doctor, but instead draws on observations and conversations with hundreds of doctors over a twenty-year period. And whilst other books involve doctors writing about their patients, in this book the mirror is reversed: doctors like Leo come to see me, a psychologist, and I am writing about them.

*

So what did happen to Leo?

With the tragic cases of students and junior doctors who had committed suicide in mind, I responded to Leo's email with considerable care. I wanted to acknowledge his obvious distress yet at the same time convey hope. I told him about other medical students and junior doctors I had encountered in the past who had expressed similar feelings. I also told him that some of them had gone on to have successful careers within medicine, whilst others had decided to build their careers outside the profession. But above all else, I emphasised that he shouldn't attempt to soldier on without help. His first priority was to go and see his GP and tell her how he was feeling. In addition, he might find it helpful to seek support from the university counselling service, as well as pastoral staff within the medical school. And I flagged up the 24-hour crisis line operated by the British Medical Association.

I explained that I was out of the country but would respond to any emails he sent me, and would be happy to talk on my return to the UK the following week. A couple of days later Leo wrote back. He'd already made contact with his GP and his personal tutor and he had found it helpful to know that I had supported other doctors who felt as he did. He also wanted to arrange a time to talk when I was back in the UK.

The following week, we talked on the phone for over an hour. Leo told me that he was feeling better than when he had first emailed me; he had contacted the BMA helpline and in addition, his GP and personal tutor had been helpful. When I asked about the impending exams Leo was clear that he was well enough to sit finals and he'd done enough studying to pass. It wasn't the exams per se that he was worried about; more what came next. When we then discussed how he felt about starting work Leo was adamant that he wanted to give it a try even if he decided a few months down the line that clinical medicine wasn't right for him.

After his exams Leo was due to go away on holiday for a month with his girlfriend. On his return he would be moving to a new town with her, to start his first job as a doctor. We left it that Leo would get in contact with me if he wanted to think about which specialty might work best for him, or if he wanted to consider leaving medicine entirely. But a couple of weeks before finals wasn't the right time to discuss either of these issues.

A month into his first job I received another email – very different from the first.

> I am happy to tell you that things got a lot better after speaking with you. I managed to pass finals and had a very relaxing holiday and have now moved in with my girlfriend. I'm working at the university hospital which is going much better than expected, and I have actually enjoyed the acute side of medicine. Anyway, I am taking things slow and steady and making sure I prioritise my own health and happiness first, and I'm trying to keep myself as balanced as I can.

It's probably a bit too early to tell how Leo's medical career will pan out in the longer term. But later on in the book we'll meet doctors who walked out within days of starting their first job; the fact that Leo is enjoying work is certainly encouraging.

I'm still shocked, however, by how frequently medical students and junior doctors find themselves at the 'edge'. Aren't there better ways of training our future doctors? Ways that mean they don't need to phone 24-hour helplines, or send desperate emails to unknown psychologists, in the hope that someone out there will listen. And couldn't we manage the transition from medical student to junior doctor better?

That's the place where these stories begin.

I

Wednesday's Child

———————————

I always ask clients about their first job as a doctor. I don't specifically ask about the first day of that first job – but sometimes, as with Hilary, that's the story I am told.

Hilary, a qualified GP, came to see me because she was thinking about leaving medicine.

'I've reached the end of the road with general practice,' she explained in our initial phone conversation.

'The only thing that I like about it is that it provides a regular income,' she continued.

Like other GPs who have come to see me, Hilary told me how she felt that contemporary general practice pulls doctors in opposing directions. On the one hand, she lived in fear of incorrectly reassuring a patient that a particular symptom didn't warrant a referral to a specialist for further investigation. On the other hand, she dreaded being singled out by her clinical managers as having an inappropriately high referral rate to specialist services. Damned if you do and damned if you don't, with no wriggle room in between.

It was five years since she had first qualified as a GP, but even before she finished her GP training, she had started to doubt whether it was the right career for her.

'I'm not a natural doctor,' she said. 'I constantly feel like a square peg in a round hole.'

But leaving wasn't easy either. Neither of her parents had been to university, and her mother's father had worked as a gardener for the local doctor.

'My mother is so proud of me, and everything that I've achieved. She really doesn't want me to change career.'

I asked Hilary to tell me about her first job as a doctor and she described how her heart sank when she saw from her rota that she'd been placed on the on-call team on her first day. What this meant was that in addition to her responsibilities on the surgical ward to which she had been attached, she also had to assess new patients as they were admitted to the hospital for surgery. It's a bit like trying to be in two places at once; nobody wants to be on call on Day 1.

On her first morning as she walked on to the surgical ward she was immediately informed by the senior nurse that, following surgery, one of the patients was extremely sick and urgently needed to be seen by a doctor. Naïvely, Hilary asked which other doctors were available.

'Mr Baker the surgical consultant is on a course, Mr Shah the registrar is on annual leave and Dr Glover is off having worked a bunch of nights. It's just you,' said the nurse.

Hurriedly, the nurse led Hilary to the patient's bedside. The first thing that Hilary clocked was the patient's strange, grey pallor. With extreme difficulty the patient opened her eyes and whispered, 'Doctor, am I going to die?' Then, a second later, a barely audible request: 'Doctor, please call my family.'

Hilary didn't have a clue whether the patient was at death's door, or whether she should urgently summon the family. More importantly, she also didn't know whether there were medical interventions she should be making, to save the patient's life. Moving away from the patient's bedside in order to confer with the nurse, Hilary asked for help.

'You're going to have to get used to this,' said the nurse. 'Mr Baker never turns down an opportunity to operate – he'll operate on anybody. With some of the patients on this ward it might have been better if they had escaped the knife. They're often even sicker when they come out of theatre.'

A junior nursing assistant called the senior nurse away. Left on her own and unsure what to do next, Hilary decided to review the patient's notes. There were no clues there either. With mounting anxiety, she wondered whether she should call the registrar from another team, or ask the senior nurse to return to the bedside. Nothing that she had learnt in medical school had prepared her for this situation.

By chance Fiona, a fledgling doctor attached to another ward, walked down the corridor and out of the corner of her eye caught sight of a panic-stricken Hilary. Realising that all was not well with her colleague, Fiona slipped away from her own clinical team, and walked on to Hilary's ward:

'Are you OK?' asked Fiona.

'Not really,' Hilary replied. 'I'm the only doctor on this ward, all the others are away today, and there's a really sick patient who looks like she is going to die.'

She led Fiona to the patient's bedside; neither of them spoke as they peered down at the sickly looking patient, who had fallen asleep again.

'I'll call my mum,' Fiona whispered.

For a second, Hilary thought that Fiona was joking. Even though she would love to magic her own mum on to the ward, she couldn't see how the appearance of Fiona's mum was going to improve the situation.

'Mum's a nurse on the Rapid Response Team,' Fiona explained. 'She'll know what to do, and I am sure she will come if I ask.'

So that's what they did. Fiona's mum was summoned and five minutes later appeared. She took one look at the patient, realised she was desperately unwell, and called the consultant anaesthetist. A couple of minutes later the anaesthetist appeared, agreed with his nursing colleague's opinion and less than ten minutes after that, the patient was transferred to the High Dependency Unit, for urgent medical treatment.

The patient survived. And Hilary's first day continued.

All the time that Hilary had been trying to sort out the desperately ill patient, her bleep had been going off, summoning her to the Surgical Assessment Unit (SAU). As soon as the patient was transferred, she dashed down to the SAU and encountered an extremely angry nurse.

'There are nine patients waiting. Where have you been?'

Before Hilary had the opportunity to explain that she had been dealing with an emergency on the ward, the nurse gave a rushed account of each of the nine patients whose names were on the whiteboard by the nursing station. Hilary absorbed almost nothing of this informational deluge.

'Is there another doctor here?' she asked, finding it hard to believe that she had been expected to fly solo on the SAU as well as on the ward.

'Triple A emergency admission.* Everyone's in theatre,' was the unwelcome response.

By this stage in the day, the nine names on the whiteboard were swimming in front of Hilary's eyes. And having already dealt with a clinical emergency (albeit by calling Fiona's mum), she was desperate to know if any of the names were higher priority than the others.

'Could you possibly help me work out who I should see first?' asked Hilary.

'Figure it out yourself, blue eyes,' was the nurse's response. And with that, she walked off – probably to get on with her own enormous list of tasks.

Over a decade had passed when Hilary told me about her Day 1, but she could still remember the face of the desperately ill patient, and her name. She could still recall that sense of panic and fear. I asked if she thought there was any relationship between her horrendous first day and her current feelings about her work; she told me that she couldn't see a link. The following day Hilary emailed me:

I was thinking yesterday about your question as to whether that first day set up any future feelings about my job and I said

---

* Triple A stands for abdominal aortic aneurysm – a swelling in the abdominal aorta, the main blood vessel that leads away from the heart, down through the abdomen, to the rest of the body. If the aneurysm bursts it causes huge internal bleeding and is usually fatal. A burst triple A is a clinical emergency.

I didn't think so. On reflection, I think that it was just the beginning of a huge number of experiences (of myself and others) that brought me to my current belief on working within NHS medicine:

That it just doesn't care. That it chews people up, spits them out and then gets another well-meaning chump to replace them. Sorry if that sounds harsh and I do have some sadness in writing it but I also think it's 100% true.

So for Hilary at least, that first day may have paved the way for extreme job dissatisfaction, ten years down the line. What strikes me most forcefully about Hilary's story is that the whole set-up seems so precarious. In the UK all first year doctors start work on the same day – the first Wednesday in August. Given that Day 1 is a national fixture across the whole country, why was the supervising consultant away on a course? Why had the registrar been allowed to go on annual leave at the same time? What if the patient had died, and Hilary had been held responsible? Why hadn't back-up provision been made on the Surgical Assessment Unit in case all the experienced staff had to rush into theatre to deal with an emergency?

Do we really want a system where a patient's life depends upon someone's mum arriving in time?

*

It would be reassuring to think that Hilary's experience was exceptional. Sadly, this is not the case. I was shocked by Hilary's conclusion that her experience was in fact commonplace. 'Lots of my F1 colleagues had similar experiences,' she told me. 'And the following year in a completely different hospital, the same thing happened to the F1 on my new team. That day I had induction in the morning into my new role as an F2 and only got to the wards in the early afternoon. But the new F1 in the team had been left to fire-fight all morning. It happens all the time.'

This conclusion of Hilary's is borne out by studies of first year foundation doctors. In fact a 2014 programme of research commissioned by the GMC reached the following conclusions:

The August transition was highlighted in our interview and audio-diary data where F1s felt unprepared, particularly for the step-change in responsibility, workload, degree of multi-tasking and understanding where to go for help . . . trainees were reasonably well prepared for history taking and full physical examinations, but mostly unprepared for adopting an holistic understanding of the patient, involving patients in their care, safe and legal prescribing, diagnosing and managing complex clinical conditions and providing immediate care in medical emergencies.

The study also emphasised how pressures on the healthcare system can impact on a recent medical graduate:

Trainees may feel prepared for situations when all goes to plan, but unprepared when exposed to high volumes of work which demand prioritization and multitasking; or uncertain thresholds (not knowing when to refer to seniors); inadequate team-working; or when seniors are not easily accessible.

*

This isn't only a pretty accurate description of Hilary's first day. Given the current pressures in the NHS, a high volume of work requiring prioritisation and multitasking has become the norm.

*

In UK hospitals it might be 'all change' on the first Wednesday in August, but the process of applying for one's first job as a doctor takes the best part of a year. Nine months earlier, in October, final year medical students fill in an online application form in which they have to rank their preference for each of the twenty-one different health regions across the whole of the UK. Jobs are allocated in score order, so the higher your score, the more likely you are to be allocated to your first or second preference region.

Each applicant's overall score comes from two separate sources. First, there is an Educational Performance Measure derived from a student's academic scores in medical school together with extra points for additional degrees and academic publications. Secondly, and given equal weight, is their score on the so-called 'Situational Judgement Test' (SJT). This is a pencil and paper test lasting over two hours during which students have to answer seventy questions. The questions are not testing clinical knowledge (that's assessed by medical school finals) but instead assess whether the applicant possesses the professional attributes needed to manage the everyday situations they may encounter in their first year of practice. For example, applicants might be given the following brief scenario:

Mr Farmer has been a patient on the ward for six months; he breathes with the aid of a ventilator following a traumatic brain injury. As you make your rounds, you notice Mr Farmer appears to be experiencing breathing problems. Both the consultant and the registrar (more senior trainee) from your team are dealing with a patient on the neighbouring ward. This is your first week and you have not yet attended a potentially critically unwell patient by yourself.

Applicants would then have to rank-order the appropriateness of the following actions in response to this situation (1 = Most appropriate; 5 = Least appropriate).

A. Call the crash team to attend to Mr Farmer as a matter of urgency.
B. Seek advice from the physiotherapy team who are on the ward and have experience in managing Mr Farmer's case.
C. Contact another registrar to discuss Mr Farmer's symptoms.
D. Ask the ward nurse to fully assess Mr Farmer's status with you immediately.
E. Ask the consultant to return to your ward straight away to attend to Mr Farmer.

The worked examples on the UK Foundation Programme Office website gives the answer as DCBEA, using this rationale:

This question is assessing your ability to make appropriate decisions in a pressurised situation. It is important to assess Mr

Farmer's status immediately. The ward nurse is most likely to be the health professional available to help and have the skills, knowledge and ability to access help if needed. It is important not to 'go it alone' if possible as help is likely to be required (D). Assessing the status of the patient should be your immediate priority and discussion with a senior colleague (C) could help reach an outcome for the patient. It can be important to have wider team involvement and informing them of patient progress is important (B). However, this would not be an immediate action and is less direct than Options D and C. Consultant return may not be appropriate until the patient is properly assessed (E). Crash teams should only be called in the case of arrest or emergency, doing otherwise could put other patients' lives at risk and is therefore the least appropriate option (A).

(Isn't it ironic that the model answer stresses the importance of asking the nurse? This is exactly what Hilary did on the Surgical Assessment Unit, only to be told that she needed to 'figure out' the answer herself. The nurse was too busy to help Hilary.)

Applicants with extremely low SJT scores have to attend a face-to-face interview, to assess whether they are competent to start working as a junior doctor. In 2016 this happened to twenty-two UK medical students and fourteen from outside the UK – only three of whom were later reinstated and offered an F1 post.

I might have struggled to believe that *anybody* could get to the end of a five- or six-year medical degree, pass finals, but lack the professional understanding to get an adequate mark on the SJT. Once one has grasped a few basic principles (patient safety always takes precedence; respect the expertise of other healthcare professionals; honesty is of the utmost importance) it seems possible to work one's way through the questions and get a reasonable score. However, when running a workshop for senior medical school faculty in one of the most academic universities in the country, an experienced clinician told me about a final year medical student who was academically brilliant, but seemed to lack sound professional judgement. On one occasion, while on an A & E placement, this particular student had needed to get his attendance form signed by the supervising consultant, but the consultant was otherwise engaged – dealing with an emergency patient resuscitation, in fact. Undeterred, the student attempted to interrupt the resuscitation, waving the form under the consultant's nose in order to get it signed.

'Should I be worried about this student?' asked the senior faculty member.

I was speechless. How could one not be worried by this student's behaviour? Isn't it fairly obvious that anybody who decides that getting a form signed takes priority over an emergency resuscitation is going to find the day-to-day demands of clinical practice impossible? Years ago, it was left to supervising clinicians to weed such students out and there can be considerable reluctance to do so, particularly if the students are academically gifted. Nowadays this task is aided by the SJT.

Final year students sit the SJT in December, and this score is added to the Educational Performance Measure to calculate their overall score. In March they are told which region they have been allocated to, or if they have been placed on the reserve list. In April they get told which specific hospital within the region they will be working at. However, those on the reserve list may not be told if a place has become available for them until right before the fateful first Wednesday in August. Between March and August medical students on the reserve list have to sit it out and wait.

What this tends to mean in practice is that the weakest final year students (those who have scored poorly on either or both of the measures) are allocated to the places which other more highly ranked students have avoided. Final year medical students can easily find out which are the less desirable posts by looking at the results from the GMC trainee surveys, alongside a host of other websites. So medical students can find out how well supported foundation doctors have felt in each of the different regions or how favourably the quality of training was rated. More highly ranked students are likely to choose those programmes where students felt better supported and better trained, whilst weaker students are left to take whatever is left over.

And there's more. Medical students can be sent to hospitals anywhere in the country – from Cornwall up to northern Scotland or Northern Ireland. Because weaker students on the reserve list will be placed in left-over slots, they are more likely to end up working in parts of the country where they know absolutely nobody, and have no accessible systems of support. This is an educational variant of what GP Dr Julian Tudor-Hart famously termed the 'inverse care law' – those who most need care, end up receiving the least. Except in this situation it isn't vulnerable patients receiving the poorest medical care – it's vulnerable medical students being offered the least support in their first post.

On paper, at least, there is a system in which final year medical students can apply to be allocated to a specific foundation programme, based on their 'special circumstances'. So, for example, if you have a school-aged child, or if you are the primary carer for somebody with a disability you can request that you won't be sent all over the country, but will be pre-allocated to a specific post. This is all good in theory, but in practice, given the stigma attached to mental health issues and the unwillingness to be seen to be struggling, very few students request this option for mental health or educational reasons.

For the last few years when the allocations have been announced in March, a small number of students have been placed on the reserve list. This always generates a lot of column space in the medical press. But in 2016 it happened to the grand number of thirty-six UK students. Tiny numbers. And by the time the programme started in August, all thirty-six of these students had been allocated jobs. In the UK, if a final year medical student passes finals (and the overwhelming majority do), and doesn't score too drastically on the SJT (which also only involves a tiny number of students) they will end up with an F1 job somewhere. It may be far from home, and it may not be one that they want – but it will be a job.

*

In the US, as in the UK, the overwhelming majority of final year medical students are offered a first year post – a residency.

For example, in 2016, less than 7% of US medical students failed to be offered a post through the National Resident Matching Program (NRMP). But there are also some key differences between the US and the UK.

First, as with so many medically related comparisons, there is the huge issue of money. UK medical students don't pay to apply to the foundation programme, whereas in the US the application for residency is anything but free. I asked a friend's daughter, Sophie, who successfully applied in 2016 for an obstetrics and gynaecology residency programme, to give me some idea of the costs, and this is what she told me:

Application fees for 55 programmes – $1,900
Transcript fees – $1,000
Fee to the NRMP – $65
Travel and hotel costs to attend 23 interviews – $6,000

So in all, Sophie reckoned that she had spent around $9,000 – a huge sum on top of an already enormous medical school debt.

Another key difference between the UK and the US is the sheer scale of the enterprise. In the US in 2016, over 30,000 residency slots were up for grabs – a figure which is more than four times greater than the number of first year posts on offer in the UK. The NRMP matches the applicants to this vast number of posts through the use of a complex mathematical algorithm which gained its two inventors – Lloyd Shapley and Alvin E. Roth – the Nobel Prize in Economics in 2012.

Prior to using this algorithm, medical students would apply to hospitals and their preferences would be visible to the selection committees. The selectors would first look at those applicants who had ranked their hospital as their first choice. If they still had vacancies the selectors would look at applicants who had ranked them second – and so on, until all their vacancies were filled. The problem with this system was that when an applicant's ranking was visible to the selectors, those applicants who had aimed too high would be severely punished. Frequently these poor medical students would end up with one of their last choices.

Nowadays applicants interview at the hospitals *without* the hospitals knowing how high up the list the applicants had rated them. Then the preferences of all the applicants and all of the hospitals are fed into the computer at the same time and the algorithm is used to create a simultaneous match between thousands of applicants and thousands of jobs that, in theory, is less influenced by the gaming strategies inherent in the old matching method. Having said that, many applicants resent the system because each individual still ends up with only one job offer. And they hate the feeling that their future depends upon the working of a complex mathematical algorithm – even if it did win somebody a Nobel Prize.

This was certainly Sophie's experience. She recognised that with the NRMP process, applicants can't (as can happen in the UK) wind up somewhere completely out of their control as they will only be considered by the specific programmes that they ranked. But she still expressed some regret.

'Do I wish we could have the opportunity for more than one programme to ultimately make us an offer and then be allowed to choose like normal adults? Yes.'

The money side of things and the sheer scale of the operation may be different in the UK and the US. But in both countries, final year medical students end up with only one offer. They look around them and see that other professions (law, business, accountancy) don't assign people to jobs this way. And, like Sophie, they resent the lack of choice. Isn't it paradoxical, considering the burden of responsibility junior doctors are expected to bear as soon as they start working, that the application system in both countries manages to infantilise final year medical students?

*

For T.S. Eliot in his epic poem, *The Waste Land*, April is the cruellest month of the year. But April is not so bad in 'Wardland' – in that realm, the calendar shifts on a couple of months and you have to worry about July and August. These are the months when medical students metamorphose into junior doctors and take up their first jobs. The jobs that they had spent the best part of the previous year applying for.

'Why July matters' is the title of a recent commentary in the American journal *Academic Medicine*. The author quotes a systematic review of thirty-nine separate studies that reached the following conclusion: 'Length of hospital stay, duration of procedures and hospital charges peaked during the month of July. Of note, rates of patient mortality also increased in this period.'

But it's not just in the US. The authors of the *Academic Medicine* paper go on to describe an international study which found that 'rates of fatal medication errors increased by 10% during the month of July in countries with teaching hospitals . . . the greater the proportion of teaching hospitals in a region, the greater the mortality rate from medication errors.'

The UK isn't immune to this effect either, but as change-over is the following month, the peak occurs in August rather than July. In 2009 a group of researchers at Imperial College in London published a retrospective study using hospitals admissions data over an eight-year period across the whole of England. The key question they looked at was whether in-hospital mortality was higher in the week following the first Wednesday in August than in the previous week. Only hospitals that took on trainee doctors on the first Wednesday in August each year were included.

As national data were gathered from across the whole of England, there was a sufficient sample size to adjust the calculations for confounding patient factors that may have affected the risk of death, including age, gender, socioeconomic status and the presence of other serious illnesses. Just under 300,000 patients were admitted on these two days in the years from 2000 to 2008. Of those, 151,844 were admitted on the last Wednesday in July and 147,897 on the first Wednesday in August. In total, there were 4,409 deaths in the two groups, 2,182 among those patients admitted on the last Wednesday in July and 2,227 among those patients admitted the week after. When the researchers adjusted for potential confounding factors, they found that the odds of death in the group admitted in August was 6% higher than the group admitted in July.

Two years later, in 2011, an online survey in the UK reported that 90% of physicians felt that the August transition had a significant negative impact on patient care and patient safety. Respondents highlighted the inadequacy of measures at the local level to support junior staff in their induction, and to ensure patient safety. The title of the paper was 'August is always a nightmare' – taken from a comment by one of the physicians in the survey. August is the cruellest month, it seems. At least for patients in teaching hospitals in the UK.

*

I didn't warm to Bella when I first met her. As I described how I worked with clients, I gained the distinct impression that she was somewhat contemptuous of what I was saying. By the end of the first session I realised that my initial impression was fundamentally incorrect. What I had initially taken to be disdain was actually a potent combination of shyness and wariness.

I had been asked to see Bella by her psychiatrist, who was treating her for depression. A couple of months earlier Bella had become so unwell that she was unable to continue in her first post as a junior doctor. Following a period of treatment (both psychotherapy and medication), her psychiatrist felt that she was now well enough to consider whether she wanted to resume her medical career. And that is why he had contacted me, and asked me whether I would be able to have some sessions with Bella.

Her psychiatrist told me that Bella was exceptionally able, winning prizes in both medicine and surgery at medical school. On paper, there were few indicators that she would be totally overwhelmed by the transition from medical student to F1 doctor; she wasn't one of the medical students who had needed to repeat years in medical school because of recurrent exam failure or ill health. But as I talked to Bella in the first session, it became clear that she had experienced mounting dread as the first Wednesday in August approached. She knew she lacked the confidence to assume responsibility for treating patients.

Over the years I have seen a number of junior doctors who have become so distressed in their first posts that they have had to stop work – at least for a period of time. When you explore their medical school history you find that almost without exception these doctors have had previous episodes of depression and anxiety. But these episodes may not have resulted in a psychiatric referral and been managed by a GP, or in sessions with a counsellor at the university counselling service. And this is what happened to Bella; a couple of years earlier, while doing her undergraduate research project, she had lost a considerable amount of weight, and started to have problems sleeping. Although Bella wasn't referred to a psychiatrist at this point, she had been to see her GP, who prescribed a brief course of antidepressants.

Bella told me that her undergraduate research supervisor found her annoying, and she ended up being poorly supported. Working on the research project was the first period in Bella's life when she didn't know what she needed to do in order to excel academically. Unfortunately Bella's supervisor had never before supervised a medical student's project and she was more interested in using Bella as free labour in the laboratory than helping her write up her research. Faced with an unresponsive supervisor, Bella felt desperately unsure about what to do. 'I felt on the precipice of failure,' she told me.

To be uncertain about how to write up a laboratory project is one thing; to be uncertain about what to do when faced with a sick patient quite another. If you make a mistake in your write-up, at worst, your project won't be awarded the top grade. If you make a mistake when looking after a sick patient, the worst thing that can happen is that a patient can die. A medical student who has become significantly depressed when faced with the uncertainty of writing up her research should have been identified as somebody who might be overwhelmed by the uncertainty inherent in treating patients. However, as Bella was so strong academically, her vulnerability remained undetected. (In the end she was awarded a first-class grade for her dissertation.)

Final year medical students have to complete a health declaration form which is forwarded to the hospital where they will be working in their first year. Bella told me that she remembers being uneasy when faced with the form; as the depression she experienced when working on her research project had never been formally diagnosed by a psychiatrist (although she had been prescribed antidepressants by her GP), she persuaded herself that she was under no obligation to mention it. She didn't want to be singled out as different – as vulnerable and weaker than her peers. At the same time, she knew that she was being less than truthful on the form and it added to her sense of foreboding as the first Wednesday in August approached.

An additional blow to Bella's confidence, prior to starting the foundation programme, was that she scored far lower than predicted on her SJT. 'If the questions assess a candidate's professional competence to handle the everyday situations that F1 doctors typically encounter, what does it say about *my* competence, that I didn't do that well?' Bella asked herself. Her lower than expected (although still average) results added to her sense of mounting dread. A more responsive (and responsible) medical school system might have picked up on the marked difference between her academic performance (where she excelled) and her SJT scores. The latter test maps more closely on to the complexity of day-to-day clinical practice. But nobody other than Bella herself foresaw a difficulty. And on a practical level, her SJT results meant that she didn't get placed in her first choice foundation programme, but instead was allocated to another part of the country where she knew nobody. The inverse care law in action.

Of course, final year medical students aren't expected to morph into first year doctors without *any* formal support. Over the last few years all medical students in the UK have been paid to shadow the doctor whose job they are going to be taking over, for a couple of days prior to the August start. Many medical schools also run 'transition to practice' courses. Bella's medical school ran such a course, but the manager in charge of the scheme told me that attendance was appalling. Bella, being conscientious, did attend this course, but she found that there was a 'disconnect' between the primarily lecture-based sessions, and the reality of what she was gearing up to face as a working doctor.

In addition, hospitals run induction courses for new starters. But a 2014 study carried out by the GMC found that the quality of induction was highly variable. Bella felt that the induction process at her hospital spent too much time dealing with practical issues such as fire alarms and manual handling of patients; at the end she wasn't in any way reassured that she was sufficiently competent to look after patients. And the one and a half days when she was supposed to shadow the F1 doctor whose role she was about to assume were cut short because the doctor was away from work on sick leave.

In a way, Bella was a victim of her previous success. 'I was somebody who had never really struggled academically, and my academic achievements and career were a big part of my identity,' she told me. And, she continued, 'It was particularly difficult for me to feel that I was struggling.'

Bella talked movingly about how difficult she found it to trust other people, or herself, and she linked this to some traumatic experiences in her childhood. Before she even started her first job, she knew that she would find the psychological demands of clinical work challenging. Whilst she understood what she described as the 'mantra' from medical school that one should always ask for help when one isn't sure, in practice, despite the fact that her clinical knowledge and skills were excellent, even minor clinical decisions caused her considerable anxiety. In her second week at work she was on call at night and had to cover *all* the medical patients in the hospital; she struggled to know when exactly she should be bleeping her senior (who was in a different part of the hospital), and when she should manage on her own.

A month or so into her first job, when Bella was working in A & E, a patient was admitted close to the end of her thirteen-hour shift. Whilst other trainees might have busied themselves with paperwork until the shift was over, Bella started to attend to this patient. She continued treating him until he was stable and all the necessary tests had been organised. Then, exactly as she had been instructed at induction, she went to find her senior in order to ensure a safe 'handover' of the patient. Bella went by the rulebook which explicitly stated that she was not to work more than thirteen hours.

The senior, probably stressed with her own workload, reacted with fury, shouting at Bella in front of the whole team, and accused her of being irresponsible. Bella was ordered to stay for as long as it took to continue treating the patient, and ended up working a fifteen-hour shift.

'What really shocked me was that I worked so hard, and followed all the rules, but I still ended up getting shouted at,' Bella said.

Feeling too exhausted to drive home, Bella retreated to the toilet, where another colleague found her sobbing in the corner. 'I couldn't bear the fact that she found me crying,' Bella told me. After this incident, she asked to be taken off the night rota, but with her confidence in shreds, an insidious depression spiralled rapidly out of control.

Bella did exactly as she had been instructed to do in medical school – she went and asked her supervising consultant for help. And his response?

'Of course this is how you feel. You're an F1. You're a girl. You're going to be upset.'

For somebody as proud and determined as Bella, admitting to a senior that she was in difficulty was far from straightforward. 'It was a huge thing to ask for help,' she said. 'And then only to be dismissed . . . ' Bella's voice tailed off.

Ten weeks into the job, Bella was so severely depressed that she was signed off sick, and referred to the psychiatrist who later contacted me. As I slowly got to know Bella over the course of the following six months, I gained an increasing respect for her determination, bravery and openness. She was an extraordinarily impressive young woman. I also learnt that, far from being haughty, she actually struggled with an acute lack of self-confidence.

Bella never resumed her career in medicine. As is often the case, although her family were initially disappointed that she wasn't going to work as a doctor, they were actually far more concerned about her well-being, and accepted her choice. It's a couple of years now since Bella was first referred to me. Despite the fact that in our initial sessions Bella was convinced that she would never be able to hold down a responsible job, for the last eighteen months she has been employed in a demanding role in the pharmaceutical sector. Judging from our recent telephone conversation, she's no longer the severely depressed young woman who felt that she had no future and who occupied her time doing 2,000-piece jigsaw puzzles.

But Bella's case still makes me angry. How is it possible for somebody to slog their way through a six-year medical degree, do brilliantly in finals, and then last just ten weeks in their first job? What does the fact that it is nearly impossible to declare a history of previous psychological difficulties say about medical school culture? Why wasn't the discrepancy between her academic and situational judgement scores seen to be a potential 'red flag' – or her earlier dramatic weight loss, for that matter? Why do the more vulnerable trainees get sent further away from home, thereby increasing the chance that they will end up having a psychological breakdown?

How could a supervising consultant joke about Bella's obvious distress?

*

Bella was certainly not alone in finding that the transition from medical school to junior hospital doctor precipitated depression. What's more, this is not a new phenomenon; articles about depression and suicide amongst junior doctors have been buried in medical journals for over thirty years. Then, from time to time, a particular suicide catches the public imagination, and coverage migrates from medical journals to the mainstream press. This happened in early 2016 at the height of the junior doctors' strike in the UK, when Rose Polge tragically killed herself by walking into the sea. For a couple of days the mental health of junior doctors made the headlines, then shortly afterwards the news moved on, and once again the whole issue got buried.

Little has changed.

In 1983, two junior doctors asked psychologist Jenny Firth-Cozens if something could be done about the stress and depression that they saw all around them. Two first year doctors in one hospital had killed themselves in the previous month, yet no senior clinicians discussed this within their teams. It was unmentionable. This prompted Firth-Cozens to undertake a series of longitudinal studies of medical students and junior doctors.

Four years later, in 1987, Firth-Cozens reported the results of a longitudinal study of 170 first year junior doctors in the *British Medical Journal* (*BMJ*): 28% of the sample had scores on standardised questionnaires that indicated the presence of a depressive illness and ten individuals reported thoughts of suicide. 'The incidence of distress is unacceptably high in junior doctors and both they and the hospitals need to deal with the causes of distress,' Firth-Cozens concluded. Twenty years after starting the first research project, another article by Firth-Cozens in the *BMJ* lamented that not enough had been done: 'What we need is a systematic approach to the problem,' she wrote.

Roll the clock on another twelve years, and in 2015 following the suicide of two first year residents in New York City, an opinion piece in a leading medical journal listed some of the ways in which medical training increases the risk of mental illness: 'Role transition, decreased sleep, relocation resulting in fewer available support systems and feelings of isolation.'

Somewhat surprisingly, the author of this paper doesn't even comment on the nature of the work that we are asking young doctors to carry out, and how this might contribute to their distress. In the same year a major international review of fifty-four previous studies, involving over 17,000 physicians in training, was published in the *Journal of the American Medical Association*. The main finding was that the extent of depressive symptoms in trainee doctors was extraordinarily high; between a quarter and a third of the sample reported experiencing significant symptoms. The authors of the study also emphasised that because the development of depression at one point in time increases the risk of *future* depressive episodes, their findings may affect the long-term health of these doctors. An accompanying editorial reached the following conclusion: 'The personal and professional dysfunction, not to mention the suicide rate that may derive from this symptom burden, should be disturbing to the profession; these findings could be easily construed as describing a depression endemic among residents.'

This wasn't the hyperbole of a tabloid headline; it was the *Journal of the American Medical Association*.

The author of the editorial then goes on to suggest that there is a fundamental 'mismatch' between the system for training doctors and the current practice of medicine. Specifically, he argues that whilst little has changed in how we train junior doctors over the last fifty or sixty years, the delivery of medical care has altered beyond all recognition. Amongst the changes in medical practice he includes: life-prolonging and life-creating technologies that lead to unsolvable ethical dilemmas; electronic medical records and documentation requirements that encourage inaccurate and sometimes dangerous copy-and-paste shortcuts; malpractice exposure in which a high proportion of residents in some specialties are named in lawsuits before finishing their training;

short hospital stays that require protocol-driven procedural care with little opportunity for thinking and learning; online ratings of physician performance; and clinical productivity pressures on faculty members that detract from the formation of strong mentorship relationships with residents. This list is not exhaustive, and some of the changes may apply more in certain healthcare systems than others. But the basic point seems incontrovertible: in many countries, the methods of training doctors no longer matches the delivery of healthcare.

There are a few exceptions, however, where training has undergone radical transformation. In New Zealand for example, since the 1970s medical students have spent their sixth and final year as 'trainee interns'. The explicit purpose of this year is to provide a more seamless transition between being a medical student and starting to practise as a doctor. In effect, trainee interns are apprentice first year doctors. During the first five years of medical school, students' clinical knowledge and competence are assessed; in the final year it is workplace-based performance. Crucially, the focus of these posts is educational as opposed to service need. Trainee interns in New Zealand would not find themselves contending with the responsibilities that doctors like Hilary faced on her first day at work. And Bella, in our sessions, described how she wanted somebody to check her work and give her regular feedback, so that she knew she was on the right track – which is exactly what happens with the trainee interns in New Zealand.

An article published in the mid-1990s in the *BMJ* suggested that the New Zealand model might have 'much to offer' the UK training system. The system might well have helped doctors like Bella. But sadly the suggestion in the article seems to have fallen on deaf ears. The fact that trainee interns are paid 60% of the salary of a first year junior doctor whilst final year medical students in the UK are not paid a penny cannot have helped – particularly with the current pressure on healthcare budgets.

Does it work? One survey reported that at the end of the trainee intern year 92% of students felt prepared to be a doctor. The authors of the survey point out that this figure is substantially higher than the proportion of final year medical students who felt ready to work as junior doctors in the UK and in the US. Even more importantly, another study in New Zealand found that the first year doctors' scores were in the *normal* range for measures of depression, anxiety and burnout. Admittedly this was a small-scale study but the contrast with the 'depression endemic' noted in studies from the UK and US is striking.

*

Improving medical education often reminds me of solving a Rubik's cube. If you twist the cube one way in order to align the colours on the top surface, all sorts of untoward changes are probably happening on the five other sides that remain hidden from view. The controversy over junior doctors' working hours is a classic example of this Rubik's cube principle. Undoubtedly over-tired doctors are problematic, for their patients, colleagues and also, of course, for themselves. But placing restrictions on junior doctors' hours turns out not to be the perfect solution. When working hours are shortened, even though there are some obvious advantages, other sides of the medical education cube such as opportunities for training or the solidarity of the team get twisted out of shape.

In the UK, the European Working Time Directive restricts the average length of the working week to forty-eight hours. The directive was first applied to senior doctors in 1998 and applied fully to junior doctors in 2009. Five years later in 2014, a review of the available evidence concluded that limiting doctors' working hours reduced both needle-stick injuries (i.e. doctors inadvertently pricking themselves when giving an injection to a patient) and road traffic accidents caused by exhausted doctors driving home after a very long shift.

As I read about the reduction of road traffic accidents, I thought of a delightful F1 doctor who had been knocked down outside the hospital early one morning, following a long night shift. Tragically he sustained significant head injuries. Following a year in rehab, and returning to work part-time, with considerable difficulty he managed to finish his foundation training. But his training programme director confided in me that she couldn't see him passing any postgraduate exams due to his poor concentration and short-term memory. In reality, his medical career was probably over.

Any measure that reduces the risk of fatigue-related injuries should be welcomed. However, evidence on the link between the reduction of working hours and depression was much more mixed, and overall the authors of the 2014 review concluded that such a link remained unproven. What this suggests is that reducing working hours per se isn't enough to protect junior doctors from depression. In fact, reducing working hours doesn't even eliminate fatigue – a finding that emerged from a telephone survey of trainees carried out in 2014. As one trainee commented: 'There's no continuity in terms of predictability . . . you run an eight cycle rota so you've got eight weeks to get through and none of those eight weeks are the same at all . . . I think that from my side is what creates fatigue.'

*

The 2017 Nobel Prize in Physiology or Medicine was awarded to Jeffrey Hall, Michael Rosbash and Michael Young. In an opinion piece published in the *BMJ*, Michael Farquhar, a London-based sleep medicine specialist, celebrated the achievement of these prizewinning researchers:

> Hall, Rosbash and Young have beautifully demonstrated how fundamental our circadian drive is to how our bodies and brains function. We owe it to all those who work at night, for their own health and for the quality of work they do, to recognise that working against that drive is difficult.

Farquhar doesn't only write articles – he's also spearheaded an initiative in his own hospital group that is gaining momentum in other hospitals across the capital. Working with the medical director and the chief nurse, Farquhar has successfully introduced teaching on basic sleep physiology and simple strategies for improving sleep as part of mandatory induction training. Some of the strategies are extremely simple – wearing sunglasses and avoiding phones and computers when one finishes a night shift, in order to maximise the chance of falling asleep when one gets home. Others are perhaps more counter-intuitive; working at night, if one wants to drink caffeine one should do it just before one takes a 15–20 minute nap – not after the nap. Caffeine takes 15–20 minutes to take effect, so if you take it before the nap, the effect will just be kicking in at the point one wakes from the nap.

Alongside this mandatory training for individuals, working with the hospital board, Farquhar is leading a culture change across the organisation as a whole. The HALT campaign (Hungry, Angry, Late, Tired) promotes the message that breaks are an essential part of effective workforce planning. Managers are tasked with leading by example; encouraging a team-based approach so that staff don't work longer than five hours at a stretch without a 15–20-minute break, identifying suitable rest areas and promoting a 'take a break' culture within the team.

One of the strands of the HALT campaign is effective rota planning – minimising frequent changes between day and night shifts. And in Farquhar's induction teaching he advises junior doctors to try, wherever possible, to minimise changes day on day as to when one goes to sleep and when one gets up. The trainee in that 2014 survey who commented on the lack of predictability of the eight-week cycle is a case in point. Rotas of this nature are precisely what sleep experts advise should be avoided. And Farquhar's campaign is a rare example of an evidence-based training intervention; knowledge gained from his clinical role as a specialist in sleep medicine is applied not just to patients, but also to the doctors and nurses who are tasked with treating these patients.

*

Of course reducing the hours that each trainee is allowed to work and campaigning that staff have regular breaks doesn't magically reduce the actual clinical tasks that need to be completed. There is still the same number of sick patients on the ward or waiting in A & E. Often working-hour restrictions exist on paper rather than in reality; the 2016 annual trainee survey carried out by the GMC found that more than 50% of doctors in training worked beyond their rostered hours on a weekly basis. This is exactly what happened to Bella. On paper she shouldn't have been working for fifteen hours on the day that it all became unbearable. But she couldn't complete all the tasks that had been allocated to her, so she just kept on going.

Not only do patients' needs stay the same, irrespective of government rulings on working hours – but juniors also have to reach the same standards of proficiency without any increase in the length of training. Particularly with the so-called 'craft' specialties such as surgery, where hands-on procedures take time to be mastered, it can be problematic to squeeze the same amount of learning into a significantly curtailed time frame.

In Britain, a government review commissioned by the Secretary of State for Health attempted to look at this very issue. But in an ironic twist that verges on the absurd – the scope of the review itself was limited by its own short time frame. (The review reported in 2010, a year on from the full implementation of the 48-hour limit on junior doctors' hours.

Given that specialty training takes at least eight years after leaving medical school, the review couldn't draw conclusions about the impact of reduced training hours on the future competency of consultants, *one* year after the working hours directive was implemented.)

What the review did find, however, was that the working hours' restrictions meant that trainees were often called in at short notice to fill gaps in the rota, particularly in evening and night shifts. During these time periods consultants are frequently not on-site, and therefore the learning opportunities are reduced. In addition, trainees often felt poorly supported at night – which is exactly what Bella, and Hilary, and a hundred other trainees have told me. The review concluded that if consultants were more directly involved in out-of-hours work, it would be possible to maintain high-quality training during the compressed timescale. But that's a big 'if'.

There's some evidence that more recent groups of trainees welcome the working hours' restrictions, and that female trainees are more positive than their male counterparts. But what is absolutely clear is that reducing the working hours hasn't solved the problem of fatigue, depression and burnout amongst junior doctors. And it might even have inadvertently compromised training in some specialties as well.

From a psychological viewpoint, probably the most significant effect of the reduction in working hours has been its impact on the so-called 'firm'. This is the old-style hierarchical working arrangement in which fledgling doctors belonged to a distinct clinical unit headed up by a consultant and supported by a number of other trainees of varying levels of seniority.

Of course this arrangement wasn't perfect; if you had a bullying or unpleasant consultant or senior registrar, your life could be made a misery. But at its best, it provided a degree of consistent psychological support for the most junior members of the team. As psychiatrist Gwen Adshead has noted, the particular language used to describe these systems – referring to them as 'attachments' or 'firms' – reminds us of their potential for providing psychological support.

Unfortunately, the move to a revolving shift system (prompted by the working hours' reduction) has disrupted the continuity of the firm. Juniors are now supervised by a changing raft of senior doctors, rather than being members of a stable team. In addition, the introduction in 2005 of three placements each of four months (as opposed to two placements of six months) has made it harder for foundation doctors; instead of having to find their place in two teams each year, they now have to settle into three.

*

In 1984 a young woman named Libby Zion was admitted to a hospital in New York City complaining of a fever and earache. Six hours after admission she was dead, due to a rare interaction between drugs she had taken prior to admission, and drugs that were administered in the hospital. Following Libby's death, her father, who was a *New York Times* journalist, campaigned for a full investigation into what had happened. The Grand Jury brought no criminal charges against the two junior doctors concerned – instead they indicted a medical education system that had allowed the error to occur.

It took nineteen years, in the States, from Libby Zion's death, for any limits on residents' duty hours to be brought into effect. Finally in 2003, a weekly limit of eighty hours was imposed. Further limits were implemented in 2011, restricting first year residents to working no more than sixteen hours in one day.

In Denmark a normal week for trainee doctors is thirty-seven hours. That's less than half the hours that trainees work in the US, *after* the restrictions were put into place in 2003. A systematic review of 135 studies on the impact on surgical trainees in the US of this so-called 'reduction' (so-called, because eighty hours per week still seems an excessive number of hours to me) found that levels of depression and burnout decreased. However, no comparable benefit was found when the daily maximum was reduced to sixteen hours. In fact there is some evidence that the sixteen-hour restrictions may have increased the rates of post-surgical complications in patients. Counter-intuitive as it at first seems, this finding can be accounted for by the fact that when doctors work shorter hours, the frequency of patient 'handover' increases.

There's an almost poetic parallel here. At the point when a medical student becomes a fledgling doctor they are transferred (handed over) from the medical school to the hospital. When this transfer happens, uncertainty, confusion and difficulties can arise on the part of the junior doctor. And so it is with patients. Doctors working shorter hours means that the care of an individual patient has to be 'handed over' more frequently between different clinical teams; that's the weak point in the system, the point at which error can creep in.

Transitions, it seems, cause trouble.

2

Finding the Middle

Cotton is not known for its soundproofing qualities. But that's all that separates one patient from their neighbour, on some hospital wards. Just a flimsy cotton curtain.

I've heard terrible things discussed on the other side of the curtain. It's a bit like toddlers playing hide-and-seek who believe that if they cover their eyes and can't see you, then you can't see them. Some doctors on a ward round who can't see the patient (because they are on the other side of a drawn curtain) act as if the patient can't hear them, or is oblivious to their presence. In reality, the patient and their family members on the other side, together with any other nearby patients, all get to hear much of the clinical team's discussion.

I can remember an elderly gentleman well into his nineties, who looked as if he was standing to attention next to his bed in a geriatrics ward. I was puzzled by the formality of what he was wearing: crisply ironed shirt, tie, sports jacket with neatly folded handkerchief in his breast pocket and smart trousers. It was almost as if he was heading off to work. The consultant asked him a couple of questions about how he had been over the previous day and night, then the team left the bedside, closed the curtain, and waited for the consultant to speak.

'That patient used to be a local GP – Dr Williams. I think he has become somewhat confused. Nurse said that he had been incontinent of urine during the night, but he didn't seem to have any memory of that at all.'

All the ward could hear this discussion.

I wasn't convinced that Dr Williams was confused. Having witnessed the conversation, my overriding sense was that the last thing in the world Dr Williams wanted to talk about, in the hearing of the rest of the ward, was his urinary incontinence. This poor man had found himself admitted to the local hospital where once he would have referred his own patients. His dress and demeanour spoke of a desperate attempt to hang on to the last vestiges of dignity. And unless he was far deafer than he seemed to be when talking to the consultant, he would have heard much of what the team said about him on the other side of the curtain.

One of my main aims when I observed these sorts of ward rounds was to encourage consultants to have a pre-ward round meeting outside the actual ward. There were so many advantages with beginning in this way: sensitive issues could be discussed out of the earshot of patients or family members, consultants could test medical students' and junior doctors' knowledge without running the risk of undermining them in front of patients, and juniors could ask questions without making patients feel that the doctors looking after them (who tend to be junior team members) didn't know what they were doing. Following this pre-meeting, the team could then go to the patient's bedside, if necessary examine the patient, and then focus on answering any questions that the patient or their relatives had about current or future clinical plans.

Over the decade that I observed doctors on ward rounds there was a gradual shift towards keeping the discussions round the bed to a minimum, coupled with greater awareness of the need to avoid sensitive conversations in places where the team could be overheard. People began to realise that the curtain round the bed was just a curtain.

One morning I turned up to do my first observation of a consultant paediatrician in another district general hospital. The team was assembled in a side room where they were holding their pre-meeting, prior to going on to the ward and seeing the actual patients. The purpose of this pre-meeting was for the junior paediatricians to discuss how each of the patients had been progressing since the consultant had last seen them, the previous day. In addition to the lead consultant, Ellen, there were three other members of the team: Suzy, a senior registrar, who was a couple of years away from completing her training in paediatrics; Ben, a senior house officer (SHO) who had two or three years' post-medical-school experience, and Vartika, a trust grade doctor, who had recently arrived in the UK from India. The crucial difference between Vartika and the two other junior team members was that her trust grade post wouldn't enable her to progress up the training ladder. Trust grade doctors are there to deliver a clinical service, and there is minimal opportunity for training built into the post. In terms of the clinical hierarchy, doctors in trust grade posts are at the bottom of the pile.

'Let's get cracking,' Ellen said. 'We'll begin reviewing whoever is in the first bay on Dolphin Ward.'

With notes in front of him, Ben started to describe Kirsty, an eight-year-old patient with diabetes who had been admitted a couple of nights previously suffering from diabetic ketoacidosis (DKA). For patients with diabetes, DKA occurs when, due to a severe lack of insulin, glucose cannot be transported from the bloodstream into the cells of the body. In the absence of glucose, these body cells start to use fat as an alternative energy source, and ketones (which alter the pH of the blood) are a by-product of this process. DKA can be life-threatening, and it happens particularly fast in children. Prompt treatment is needed, with a closely monitored mixture of insulin, glucose and intravenous fluids. When Kirsty was admitted she was unconscious, but three days later her blood glucose levels had been stabilised and she was well enough to be discharged.

'Good,' said the consultant. 'That's pretty straightforward. Who's next?'

Ben opened a second set of notes, and started summarising the clinical history of Jack, a six-month-old baby, who had been in hospital for a couple of days with severe breathing difficulties. Jack had been diagnosed as suffering from bronchiolitis, an acute inflammation of the small airways in the lungs. Three days ago his frantic parents had called an ambulance when it looked to them as if their baby was stopping breathing entirely. The ambulance took him to A & E and he was admitted on to the paediatric ward very quickly. In the couple of days prior to this hospital admission he had seemed very miserable with a hacking cough, a severely blocked-up nose, and difficulty feeding.

'How's he been overnight?' Ellen asked.

'Much better, his oxygen sats are now fine.'

'Well, let's take him off the oxygen and see how he does. With a bit of luck he should be home in a couple of days. Anybody else we need to discuss?'

Ben described a ten-year-old patient, Jasmine, who had been admitted overnight with a high fever. Swabs had been sent off to the pathology lab but the results weren't ready yet, so the source of infection hadn't been established.

'I wonder if it's tonsillitis,' Ellen commented.

'We tried to look at her throat in A & E, but Jasmine didn't want to play ball.'

'OK, we'll take a look now.'

And so the pre-meeting went on for the next quarter of an hour. Ben reviewed the notes of the other children on the ward and the consultant briefly commented on how she thought the patients were progressing, other clinical investigations that needed to be carried out, and when it might be safe for the children to be discharged. An unmemorable pre-meeting, in an equally unmemorable small district general hospital. Nothing prepared me for what happened next.

As soon as Ben had worked his way through all the notes, Ellen informed the team that the ambulance service had been called to a house in the local town at five o'clock that morning. A couple had put their four-month-old baby son to bed at ten o'clock the previous night. When he failed to wake for his regular early morning feed the mother went into his bedroom, and couldn't rouse him. The ambulance quickly arrived on the scene – but tragically the baby was pronounced dead. The parents, together with the body of their baby, were brought into hospital. Nursing staff were with the parents, and the chaplain had been called. But somebody from the paediatric team needed to go and formally certify the death.

Ellen turned to Suzy, who immediately responded by saying that she wasn't on call for emergencies. They both then turned towards Ben who was the next most experienced doctor in the pecking order.

'It's not my turn either, to be on call.'

All three then stared at the only remaining person in the room – Vartika. The bottom of the medical pile.

'I don't know how to certify a baby's death,' Vartika responded. 'I've never done that before in the UK and I've only been in the country a few weeks.'

As quickly as this task had been passed down the chain of command (from consultant, to registrar, to SHO, to trust doctor), it went back up again. None of the others seemed to have heard what Vartika had said, and instead were quick to give reassurance.

'There's a protocol in the file,' said Ben.

'The files are at the nurses' station,' said Suzy.

'It's quite straightforward,' said Ellen.

'I'm really not sure how this is done,' Vartika repeated. 'Death certification might be completely different here, from how I did it in India.'

Once again, the same reassurance was passed down the food chain, with the other three doctors reiterating that it really wasn't difficult and anyway, all the instructions were in the file.

'If you've got any queries, ring the ward,' Ellen said. 'It won't take you too long. When you are finished, come and join us.'

And with that Ellen, Suzy and Ben left. Vartika remained standing in the middle of the room, barely moving, with a terrified look on her face. I noted this down on my observation sheet, attempted to give her a reassuring smile and then followed the rest of the team as they walked round the corner to the paediatric ward.

First stop on the ward round was Kirsty, the eight-year-old girl who had been admitted a couple of days previously with diabetic ketoacidosis. She was sitting up in bed playing an electronic game and didn't seem at all perturbed when the three doctors walked in.

'How are you feeling today?' Ellen asked.

With reluctance Kirsty looked up from the screen. 'I'm a bit bored. Can I go home now?'

'I just need a word with your mum first,' Ellen replied, 'and then you'll be good to go.'

Ellen explained that she had asked the specialist diabetic nurse to come and see Kirsty before she was discharged, and the nurse would also give them a date for an outpatient appointment.

'Bye, Kirsty,' the three doctors chorused, and they then moved on.

The trio had just drawn back the curtain and were about to walk into the bay with the next patient, when they were interrupted by the ward sister.

'An Indian-sounding doctor is on the phone and wants to talk to you urgently,' the nurse told Ellen.

'Wait here, and I'll be back in a moment,' Ellen said as she followed the nurse out to the telephone.

A couple of minutes later Ellen returned, muttering under her breath.

'OK, shall we continue?'

The next patient was more complicated. Jack was the six-month-old baby who had been admitted a couple of days previously with breathing difficulties. Perhaps the memory of the dead baby was in everybody's mind, but for whatever reason, Jack was examined carefully from top to toe. Finally the group checked the most recent oxygen saturations in the notes at the end of his cot and it seemed as if Jack was on the mend.

'Let's try him off the oxygen,' Ellen said to Jack's mother. 'We'll see how he gets on. But I want to keep a close eye on him today, before we think of letting him home. How's he been feeding?'

'Much better,' the mother replied. 'He seems a bit more like his usual self.'

Ellen smiled. 'Let's see how his breathing is today, and we'll think about a discharge tomorrow.'

Ben and Suzy peered down into the cot and waved goodbye to Jack. Slowly he broke into a shy smile.

The third patient, Jasmine, was the ten-year-old girl who had been admitted overnight with a high fever. The group were huddled around Jasmine's bed, and the consultant was about to start examining her when the same nurse reappeared.

'Vartika on the phone for you. Again,' said the nurse.

Raising her eyes to the ceiling in a look of irritation, the consultant asked the registrar to continue the ward round.

'I'm not sure when I'll be back, but clearly Vartika can't be left on her own.'

Suzy straightened her posture and seemed pleased to be deputising for the consultant. The reduced team of two turned their attention back to Jasmine. Following the discussion in the pre-ward round meeting, Suzy knew that she needed to look inside Jasmine's mouth to examine her throat. She pulled out a tongue depressor from her pocket – an instrument that looks a bit like an overgrown ice-lolly stick. It's not particularly pleasant to have one's tongue pressed down by it, and both children and adults dislike the procedure. Paediatricians are taught to examine the throat last so that if the child is going to become distressed they can immediately be comforted, rather than having to carry on with examining another part of the body.

Suzy did everything in the correct order, leaving the throat examination till last. However, she didn't ask Jasmine's mum to hold her daughter in a firm cuddle when she introduced the tongue depressor into her mouth, and instead pushed it in with some force. Jasmine clenched her jaw around the instrument with all the strength she could muster.

'Come on, Jasmine, help me out here and open your mouth,' Suzy instructed.

Jasmine's jaw didn't relax a millimetre.

'I need to look at your throat. We need to find out why you are feeling poorly.'

Jasmine's mouth remained fixed. She stared at Suzy.

Perhaps unfairly, I'd taken something of a dislike to this registrar. She hadn't offered to support Vartika, and she hadn't been particularly gentle with Jasmine. I could tell that she was unhappy that Jasmine hadn't complied with her instructions, and she had been made to look less than competent in front of a patient, the patient's mother, a more junior doctor. And of course, in front of me.

For a moment I thought that Suzy was going to use brute force to get Jasmine to open her mouth. She then had second thoughts, and withdrew the instrument entirely.

'We'll come by a bit later, and try again,' she said.

And with that, all three of us left the ward.

My job was to observe how the consultant trained her juniors, so in the absence of the consultant, I was left without a clear role. The two juniors went off to see patients on another ward, and I waited for Ellen to return.

As I sat in the office wondering how Ellen and Vartika were getting on, my mind turned back to another paediatric ward round that I had observed years previously. Raj, the consultant on that occasion, couldn't have been more different to Ellen. He was warm, gentle and kind. I remembered how a little boy of about two or three wriggled off his mother's lap and ran away when Raj walked into his bay on the ward. The boy's parents had been mortified and shouted to him, but Raj had simply followed the boy to the centre of the ward where there was a large pile of toys. By crouching down next to where the boy was playing, Raj got his stethoscope out and carried out the examination while the boy was absorbed by the toys.

Later that afternoon on the same ward round, Raj was summoned to an emergency in A & E. The helicopter service had been called to an eleven-year-old boy who had been hit by a car; the boy wasn't expected to survive. Raj's registrar wanted him to come down to A & E, to talk to the boy's parents. I waited a very long time that afternoon, increasingly anxious about getting back to my own children because the observation was taking much longer than anticipated. At the same time I was acutely aware how trivial my own childcare concerns were, in comparison to the devastating information that Raj had to convey to the dead boy's parents.

Just when I had decided that I would leave Raj a note and head off home, he returned, looking exhausted. I had imagined that the last thing he would have wanted to do was to get my feedback for his ward round teaching – but I was wrong. Perhaps as a way of de-intensifying the emotional load of the day, he wanted to shift his attention from telling parents about the death of their child, to the more benign task of listening to my feedback. I had no doubt that he had been as compassionate with the bereaved parents as was humanly possible and the strain in his face showed that the encounter had taken its toll.

As with Raj, I waited a long time for Ellen to return to the ward. But unlike Raj, she didn't want to receive my feedback on the ward round and suggested that perhaps we could talk on the phone at a later date. I wasn't willing to comply with this request as I felt it was my responsibility to point out her failure to respond to Vartika's desperate requests for assistance.

There are different models of how best to give critical feedback, but none of them suggest that you should go straight for the kill. Yet that's precisely what I did with Ellen. I didn't attempt to re-establish rapport, or get her sense of what had worked well in the pre-ward round meeting. Instead I gave her copies of my observation notes and pointed out that I had noticed Vartika's distress from the moment she first said she didn't feel able to certify the baby's death. My anger at Vartika's abandonment spilled over into how I approached giving Ellen feedback. It was a poor piece of pedagogy on my part and I wasted a valuable opportunity to model a more supportive stance. Although the stakes were much lower, I failed to meet Ellen's needs in much the same way that she failed to attend to Vartika.

Ellen did allow me to come back and do the subsequent observations but our relationship never quite recovered. Despite frequent reminders, it took her nine months to agree on a date for the next session. The spectre of the dead baby, the unsupported trust grade doctor and the angry psychologist never quite went away.

*

What is it that makes some doctors empathic, and acutely attuned to the emotional needs of those around them, whilst others remain oblivious to other people's distress? Why did Ellen fail to support Vartika, whilst Raj treated everyone around him with kindness? Why did I continue the pattern of insensitivity, and compromise the support that I offered Ellen?

If I start with myself, it was my anger that got in the way, perhaps tinged with an element of shame. My role was to observe how Ellen trained her team, not to intervene in the day-to-day running of the ward round. But when we abandoned Vartika, I could have asked Ellen for a quick word, in private. I had noticed Vartika's distress but failed to assume a more active role in getting her the help she needed.

What about Ellen? Perhaps she had been on call the previous night, and was short of sleep. Or perhaps she had young children at home who had kept her up at night. It's harder to be empathic when one is exhausted; that's why reducing the working hours of junior doctors has been shown to enhance their capacity for empathy.

But it's not only exhaustion that influences our adult capacity for empathy. Despite the fact that adults typically remember little that happened to them prior to the age of three, our experiences in infancy have a pervasive impact on our psychological functioning throughout life. In particular, the quality and consistency of our early relationships with a primary carer (who doesn't have to be our mother) shapes how we tend to respond when we feel threatened by separation or loss.

These ideas are not new. In the aftermath of the Second World War, the paediatrician and psychoanalyst John Bowlby studied children who had been orphaned, and noticed the damaging impact that parental loss had on their subsequent psychological development. Bowlby then became interested in how psychological bonds (which he termed 'attachments') develop between infants and carers, why these bonds develop, and what happens when the normal process of attachment is disrupted. Drawing on research from animal behaviour, Bowlby recognised the evolutionary advantage of an infant being able to signal distress to their carer when they feel under threat, thus drawing the carer into closer proximity.

Later, Bowlby's student, Dr Mary Ainsworth, conducted a series of observational experiments (known as the 'Strange Situation'), in order to assess differences in how infants of one to two years of age were attached to their parents. These experiments took place in a playroom which was new to the infant, and full of toys. Throughout the experiment the infant was observed through a one-way mirror. A set series of events took place, with the parent leaving the room and coming back a few minutes later. Sometimes a stranger was present in the room, and sometimes not. The events were designed to be stressful enough to trigger an attachment response on behalf of the infant.

The observers behind the mirror looked closely at how the infant responded to the stranger, to the departure of the mother, and then to their later reunion with the mother. Through studying hundreds of infants in this experimental situation, Ainsworth concluded that there were three different ways in which infants can be 'attached' to their mothers. Infants who were 'securely' attached to their mothers readily explored their new surroundings when their mother was present, showed anxiety in the stranger's presence, were distressed by their mother's brief absence, rapidly sought contact and were quickly reassured once the mother returned. About 60% of infants fell into this group.

The remaining 40% of infants were classified as 'insecurely' attached and exhibited one of two different patterns of behaviour in the experimental situation. Infants whose insecure attachment was classified as 'avoidant' appeared less upset at separation, might not seek contact with the mother on her return and might not prefer the mother to the stranger. In contrast, infants whose insecure attachment was classified as 'resistant' showed limited play initially, became highly distressed by the separation and did not easily settle once the mother reappeared. A subsequent group of researchers identified a third group of insecurely attached infants with 'disorganised' attachment. This was characterised by first seeking contact from the mother on her return, but then, once they were close to the mother, becoming extremely fearful. In addition these researchers also developed a way of assessing adults' attachment – the so-called Adult Attachment Interview (AAI). This semi-structured interview consists of twenty questions and takes about one hour to administer. During the interview, participants are asked to describe early childhood experiences with primary attachment figures and evaluate the impact of these experiences on their development.

On the face of it, how infants respond to their mothers (or primary caregiver, if the person regularly looking after the infant doesn't happen to be the mother) might seem to have little to do with doctors. But studies have shown the enduring impact of our early attachment relationships on aspects of our adult life that have a direct bearing on the medical profession. Thinking first about being on the *receiving* end of medical care, the nature of the patient's early attachment experience influences how they respond to illness. For example, a 2012 study found that patients who go regularly to their GP with vague medical symptoms, which never get diagnosed, tend to have insecure attachment styles. The authors of this study concluded that these patients' high consultation rates could be thought of as a form of care-seeking behaviour, linked to their insecure attachment. Similarly, another study of terminally ill cancer patients found that those with a secure attachment style had a greater capacity to form a close working alliance with their physicians.

What is perhaps more surprising is that one's early attachment experience not only influences how we respond when we are the recipients of care, but is also implicated in our capacity to give care to others. Gwen Adshead, a forensic psychiatrist, beautifully describes how this works:

> Early attachment experience becomes represented cognitively in the brain as an 'internal working model', a complex schema of images, beliefs and attitudes towards attachment relationships ... the 'caregiver icon' which is engaged psychologically when the individual is either in need of care or has to provide it.

So how we were cared for when we were dependent infants influences our capacity to care for others, when they too are vulnerable.

*

A sick or dying baby is probably the most powerful example of a human being in need of care. From a psychological point of view, a dead baby represents a catastrophic failure of care.

There's no escaping the fact that managing one's emotional response to this situation is a demanding psychological task. On the morning that I observed the ward round, Ellen and the two other trainees didn't want to think about the dead baby, or the parents – and instead chose to dump their duties on the least powerful doctor in the room.

And it's not only the tragedy of a baby's death that imposes a psychological burden on healthcare staff. Caring for babies in the early stages of life, particularly if they have been born very prematurely, can also be an acute psychological stress for some doctors. Of course on a practical level, the physical tasks associated with medical care (taking blood samples, putting in a cannula) are much trickier when the patient is tiny. But when trainees have talked to me about their intense fear of the neonatal ward it probably has as much to do with their personal response to extreme vulnerability, as with any problems linked to tricky practical procedures. This was made clear to me when a medical student called Laura came to see me. Laura had a long history of anorexia and staff at the medical school were gravely concerned whether she was well enough to start working as a foundation doctor. Laura had opted to spend her elective period in her final year at medical school working on the paediatric wards. I didn't think it coincidental that whilst she could cope with older children in the paediatric ward, some of whom were suffering greatly, it was the neonates that she found most disturbing. The tiny, scrawny premature babies presented an image of extreme vulnerability that in some way mirrored her own physical and psychological state. I have never forgotten Laura's intense feelings about neonates and the way in which it dramatically illustrates how the needs of the patient can reverberate within the psyche of the doctor.

We also need to remember that we require young (and some-times vulnerable) doctors to carry out appallingly difficult things – like certifying the sudden and unexpected death of a baby. I asked a consultant paediatrician colleague exactly what this entailed:

Only a doctor can certify death, so this task cannot be delegated to a nurse. The doctor would probably not be alone. The parents would be given the option of attending, and if they chose to, they would probably be accompanied by a senior nurse to support them. The police have to be informed of a sudden death of a child, and they might be in attendance as well, if any aspect of the case made them concerned that a non-accidental injury had taken place.

First the doctor would check that there were no signs of life. Then they would have to remove the baby's clothes and examine their whole body, carefully documenting any find-ings. If there was any resuscitation equipment, they would note it, but leave it in place. In order to establish the cause of death, the doctor would take swabs from different parts of the body, blood and urine samples, and perhaps cerebro-spinal fluid.

If the parents requested it, a forelock of hair might be cut, for the parents to keep. Or foot and hand impressions might be taken, or a photo. Then the baby's body would be wrapped up.

Next the doctor would speak to the coroner, to discuss their findings, and a designated person within the hospital would also need to be informed. A 'Rapid Review' meeting would be convened within a couple of days, with the parents, consultant, police and social workers all present.

My paediatrician colleague was appalled that this task had been delegated to a trust grade doctor who had only recently arrived in the country. Apart from anything else, the whole issue of non-accidental injury might be thought of completely differently in the UK than in India. This colleague also said that her registrars don't learn from a protocol in a file, but instead go on a full-day training course before they would be asked to certify the death of a baby. And even after they have been taught what needs to be done, you can never escape the emotional impact of the task. As the consultant, she would want to have a quiet word with a trainee afterwards, so the trainee feels supported throughout.

Death, dying, distress and disease are inescapable components of a doctor's work. It's hard to see how it could be otherwise. Excruciatingly difficult tasks cannot be surgically removed from the daily 'to do' list of healthcare staff. What can shift, however, is our understanding of the psychological demands that carrying out this work entails.

So how do doctors (or anybody else, for that matter) respond when they hear a patient screaming in pain, or they see the ravages of disease or trauma on somebody's body. How do they manage when they need to tell a parent that their child has died? What resources can the doctor draw on in these situations?

Just as the body has a whole system of defence against infection (the immune system) which kicks into action when a pathogen is detected – so too does it have a way of protecting itself from emotional disintegration in the face of overwhelming psychological stress. In the immune system, the component parts such as the B cells, and the antibodies they produce, have an actual physical presence in the body – they can be analysed and measured in the blood. But the psychological defence system doesn't reside in a particular part of the human anatomy. Instead, as the psychiatrist and psychoanalyst George Vaillant puts it, mechanisms of defence are 'metaphors . . . not pieces of clockwork'. Crucially, Vaillant goes on to stress that defence mechanisms 'are normal responses to abnormal circumstances'.

Take avoidance – a really common defence mechanism. For whatever reason, it seems that Ellen's automatic response was to avoid having to certify the death of the baby, or having to help somebody else from the team do so. I wanted to avoid confronting Ellen with how she had treated Vartika. Laura wanted to avoid having anything to do with neonates. Often this happens automatically, and beyond our conscious awareness.

*

When I train hospital consultants in how best to support their trainees, I frequently ask them how they know if one of their junior team members is struggling. Without hesitation they reel off a list of warning signs such as frequent absence due to sickness, arriving late, leaving early, or failure to respond to their bleep. These answers are all correct, and have been well documented in the literature. What the consultants often don't see is that each of these behaviours represents an avoidant response on the part of the junior doctor. If you stay at home or you shorten the working day, you will reduce your personal exposure to experiences at work that you are finding aversive. If you fear that you will be asked to carry out clinical tasks that are beyond your level of competence, you are not going to rush to answer your bleep. These responses may be deeply unhelpful for the patient or for the other members of your team, but from a psychological point of view they make perfect sense.

Another defensive strategy is intellectualisation – concentrating on the dry, factual, intellectual bits of a situation while ignoring the possibility that it could have any impact on one's feelings. Vartika was told that everything she needed to know would be included on the pro-forma but this advice entirely missed the point. A list of instructions is ideal for putting together a piece of self-assembly furniture or guiding one through a new recipe, but it doesn't begin to address the emotional complexities of certifying the death of a baby.

The late Simon Sinclair, a psychiatrist and social anthropologist, in his observational study of medical training gives another powerful example of the ever-present pull towards intellectualisation. Sinclair describes how a mature student, following an embryology lecture in which slides of human foetuses at different stages of development were shown, commented 'I could only see them [the slides] each as personal tragedies for someone'. But as Sinclair goes on to point out, this student would have to reconceptualise what these slides represented, and use them to learn the stages of organ development, in order to pass his end-of-year examination.

And then there are the twin defensive strategies of suppression and repression. The former represents a conscious decision to delay paying attention to one's feelings in order to cope with the present reality. Doctors have to suppress their emotions all the time, when they deliver a painful or unpleasant treatment to a patient. In this situation they must focus on the provision of safe care, and may have to suppress their desire to stop inflicting pain on the patient.

Repression, in contrast to suppression, is the defensive strategy in which difficult emotions are pushed out of the conscious mind entirely. This happens in medicine, when doctors become so emotionally overloaded by different aspects of their work that they stop feeling anything at all. Physician Danielle Ofri describes a paediatric trainee at the end of her training programme, who received no support in managing the emotional consequences of treating dying children or mourning parents. Faced with a four-year-old boy in intensive care, who had suffered catastrophic brain damage after falling into a lake, the trainee told Ofri, 'I felt absolutely nothing for that boy and his family during the entire two weeks I cared for him . . . I was almost finished with residency, almost out of this mess where I was always dealing with dead or near-dead children. I was determined that this was not going to bring me down.'

What this resident is describing here is a catastrophic erosion of empathy; in the end she changed specialty because she didn't want to respond to her patients in this way. If this resident was a lone example it would be a personal problem for that doctor, and for her patients. But the situation is much more worrying than that. A recent systematic review concluded that nine out of eleven studies of medical students, and six out of seven studies of medical residents reported a consistent decline in empathy as training progressed. Some of the reasons given for this finding include sleep deprivation, excessive workload, mistreatment by superiors and lack of positive role models. In other words, the environment in which doctors work has a significant impact on their capacity to respond empathically to patients. Unfortunately, Ellen's response to Vartika, or Suzy's unsympathetic treatment of some of the in-patients on the ward are far from unique.

Yet as we'll come to see in later chapters, it's also possible to have too much empathy – to feel the patient's pain too acutely. The doctor needs the capacity to imagine the physical or psychological pain that the patient is experiencing, but mustn't be overwhelmed by the patient's suffering. So how can this be achieved?

Over a hundred years ago, the Canadian physician William Osler, in his essay *Aequanimitas*, wrote that the doctor should aspire to a form of emotional detachment such that 'his blood vessels don't constrict and his heart remains steady when he sees terrible sights'. That was the gold standard at the turn of the century. More recently in the 1960s, sociologist Renée Fox and psychiatrist Harold Leif argued that students should view the cadaver in the dissecting lab as their 'first patient' and the detachment with which they approach the task of human dissection should form a model for future interactions with live patients. According to these authors, the ideal was to develop an attitude of 'detached concern'. And as recently as 1999, a statement produced by the Society for General Internal

Medicine concluded that 'empathy is the act of correctly acknowledging the emotional state of another *without* experiencing that state oneself'.

But does detachment from all human emotion really enhance the doctor's effectiveness? Psychiatrist Jodi Halpern has researched this issue for a number of years and concluded that the rationale for 'detached concern' is no longer tenable: emotionally attuned physicians have a better understanding of their patients, and their patients are more likely to disclose sensitive information and stick to the prescribed treatment plan.

Even the notion that emotional connection with one's patients inevitably leads to doctors becoming emotionally overwhelmed isn't supported by the evidence. For example, a recent study of over 7,000 physicians found that those with greater empathic concern for their patients were more satisfied with their work than those who struggled to regulate their feelings and responded by becoming emotionally disengaged from their patients; the latter were more likely to experience burnout. Thus it seems that it's not *having* feelings that causes problems for doctors but not being able to *regulate* these feelings. (Unsurprisingly, the authors of this study also pointed out that working shifts of 36–48 hours without a break dramatically reduced doctors' capacity for emotional regulation.)

Another writer – the late Michael Crichton – gave a vivid account of this process of emotional regulation. Crichton, author of *Jurassic Park* and creator of the television series *ER*, originally trained as a doctor. In 'Medical Days' h•

described his experience of human dissection at Harvard Medical School in the 1960s:

> Somewhere inside me there was a kind of click, a shutting-off, a refusal to acknowledge in ordinary human terms what I was doing. After that click, I was all right. I cut well. Mine was the best section in the class . . .
>
> I later learned that this shutting-off click was essential to becoming a doctor. You could not function if you were over-whelmed by what was happening . . . I had to find a way to guard against what I felt.
>
> And still later I learned that the best doctors found a middle position where they were neither overwhelmed by their feelings nor estranged from them. That was the most difficult position of all, and the precise balance — neither too detached nor too caring — was something few learned.

*

In the summer of 1995, thirty or so years after Michael Crichton left Harvard Medical School, a forty-year-old man with terminal lung cancer, Kenneth Schwartz, was admitted as a patient to the hospital attached to the medical school – Massachusetts General Hospital (MGH). Schwartz was a lawyer who specialised in healthcare law, and shortly before his death he wrote about his experience of being a patient for the *Boston Globe Magazine*:

> I realize that a high-volume, high-pressure setting tends to stifle a caregiver's inherent compassion and humanity. But the

briefest pause in the frenetic pace can bring out the best in a caregiver and do much for a terrified patient. It has been a harrowing experience for me and for my family. And yet, the ordeal has been punctuated by moments of exquisite compassion. I have been the recipient of an extraordinary array of human and humane responses to my plight. These acts of kindness – the simple human touch from my caregivers – have made the unbearable bearable.

Aware of the cost-cutting pressures on healthcare delivery from his legal work, he knew how difficult it could be for staff to remain empathic:

In such a cost-conscious world, can any hospital continue to nurture those precious moments of engagement between patient and caregiver that provide hope to the patient and vital support to the healing process?

After his death, his family created a non-profit organisation dedicated to strengthening the patient–caregiver relationship. And one of the most successful initiatives devised by the organisation was the so-called 'Schwartz Center Rounds'. This started as a pilot programme at MGH in 1997, but twenty years later has been adopted by over four hundred hospitals across North America, the UK, Ireland and New Zealand.

So what is a Schwartz Center Round?

Basically it's an hour-long opportunity for staff from across the hospital – both clinical and non-clinical – to get together to discuss the difficult emotional and ethical issues that arise in their day-to-day work. Or put differently, Schwartz Rounds provide an opportunity for staff to discuss the human dimensions of care. Topics include working with a difficult patient or family; medical mistakes; breakdowns in communication; bigotry surrounding obesity; complementary and alternative therapy; spirituality. In effect – all and any of the real difficulties that hospital staff face at work.

A number of things mark Schwartz Rounds as different from other hospital-based educational initiatives: they are multidisciplinary, spanning both clinical and non-clinical staff; the thoughts, feelings and dilemmas of participants are brought to the fore rather than concentrating on narrowly clinical aspects of care; and the meetings are led by an experienced facilitator who teases out emerging themes and also ensures that everybody who wants to gets the opportunity to speak.

So do Schwartz Rounds work? Do they actually have an impact on the patient–clinician relationship, or on staff wellbeing?

Admittedly much of the evidence on the impact of Schwartz Rounds is somewhat anecdotal; as a recent study in the *BMJ* argued, 'we do not know what proportion of staff – or which staff – may need to attend Rounds (and over what period) in order to maximise the impact of this organisational innovation'.

Fair enough. But the 'anecdotal' evidence is certainly encouraging, with staff in a 2017 study making the following sort of comments:

'Very human emotional issues get discussed that perhaps we don't voice that often . . . but what has been interesting is that being voiced in a wider public forum and everybody being able to relate to it.'

'Actually seeing senior people being quite open about the impact of people whom they have worked with in the past is actually incredibly valuable.'

'I think it is very healthy to be exposed to other networks, other disciplines, other people and go, oh they have the same kind of stresses as we do . . .'

Nobody has yet published a study showing a downside to Schwartz Rounds. (I suppose one downside might be if they became a 'one size fits all' simple solution. An hour a month isn't going to solve the problem of burnout, or lack of empathy across a whole institution.) And the 2017 study also emphasised that successful implementation of the initiative requires 'strong leadership' from the top.

*

Schwartz Rounds aren't the only way that staff can be supported in the emotional demands of their work. The best clinicians have done this quite instinctively in their one-to-one and group teaching sessions. Clinicians like Bernard Heller.

The first time I met Bernard, it was to observe him teaching a lunchtime session for junior doctors in a hospital outside London. Lunchtime teaching sessions can be challenging; the speaker may not know who they are supposed to be teaching and it is perfectly possible that they have never previously met any of the medical students or junior doctors in the room. To make matters worse, they may also have little sense of what they should be teaching. Sometimes there is no curriculum that could be used as a reference point whilst at other times attendees could be at such divergent stages of training, it would be impossible to meet the educational needs of everybody present.

Then there's the issue of interruptions. Lunchtime teaching is supposed to be 'protected' time, with juniors handing over their bleeps for the duration of the session. But the protection often doesn't amount to much. Both as a teacher and as an observer, I've been in sessions where there have been over twenty bleep interruptions during the course of an hour. It's hard to keep focused on one's teaching when one is interrupted every other minute.

Juniors also finish their morning ward rounds at different times. Whilst some may be there at the start of the session, others wander in, often apologising profusely, throughout the hour. And there's the question of lunch. Sometimes it is provided, and I have been amazed by how appreciative junior doctors are when this happens. Often they bring in lunch from elsewhere. But whatever the source, the teaching session may be the only time during a long day that the juniors get to sit down and eat. The sound of rattling crisp packets and unwrapping sandwich packs is a frequent accompaniment to the voice of the presenter.

Bernard started off by introducing himself and explained that he was based at the local hospice. He then introduced me and mentioned that I was observing him and not them, and they didn't have to worry about my presence. Over the years I have been surprised how often consultants forgot to tell students or trainees that I wasn't there to judge them; taking the time to do so was often a sign that the consultant had the reflective ability to think about what was happening in the room from the learner's point of view.

Bernard put up the first slide, which showed his name and the title of the talk: 'Managing Breathlessness in End of Life Care'. He was just about to move on to the second slide when one of the juniors interrupted:

'Dr Heller, can I ask you a question, please?'

'Of course, go ahead,' Bernard answered.

'Well it's not specifically about breathlessness, but it is about end of life. Is that OK?'

Bernard responded with a nod.

'Last weekend we had this patient on Blue Ward who was dying of bowel cancer. What was really upsetting was that they were in terrible pain, and they kept on screaming and asking for help. Nobody I asked seemed to know what to do. I called the registrar, but she didn't get up to the ward before the patient died. Afterwards I asked the nurses if this often happened, and they said that it definitely wasn't a one-off.'

Bernard made sure that the junior had finished before he spoke.

'That must have been difficult for you to see. I'm glad that you brought this to my attention.

'Which team was this patient admitted under?' he asked.

The junior told him, and Bernard noted it down without comment.

'What about other wards in the hospital? Have others of you had to witness patients dying with poorly controlled pain?'

There were perhaps twenty junior doctors in the room. At least a third indicated with their hands that they too had witnessed distressing deaths.

'I want to make sure that everybody here has the opportunity, if they want, to tell me about their experience. Although these patients may be admitted through A & E, end-of-life pain relief is the responsibility of the palliative care team. I need to get a sense of what has been happening.'

Different doctors round the room told their stories. Some spoke about end-of-life care in this hospital. Others talked about previous hospitals they had worked in, where the end-of-life care was better (or, in some cases, even worse). As each junior described what they had seen, Bernard took detailed notes. On occasion he asked the junior to repeat what they had just said, in order to make sure that he had noted it down accurately.

'Anybody else like to add to the discussion?' Bernard asked.

Round the table, the juniors shook their heads.

'Thanks for listening,' one of the doctors said. 'It was good to get it off my chest.'

'This isn't only about getting things off your chest,' Bernard responded. 'There are clearly improvements that need to be made. I'm going to talk to the Foundation Programme Director, to the person who organises the medical registrars' teaching sessions, and to the Director of Nursing. I also want to go and organise some teaching for the medical on-call team. It might take some time, but I'm going to set these things up as a priority. We'd better get back to breathlessness now, as that is what we were supposed to be looking at this lunchtime.'

'Dr Heller, lots of us are going to have to leave at two on the dot. Is it worth starting your talk?'

It was now quarter to two. The look on Bernard's face indicated that he had been so absorbed by listening to the juniors, taking accurate notes and making sure that everybody who wanted to had been given a turn, that he had completely lost track of the time. He paused.

'Probably best not to start on a whole new topic at this point. Let's just call it a day.'

The juniors thanked him for listening to them and, still talking, in twos and threes left the teaching room.

When everybody had gone, Bernard turned to me.

'You're probably going to fail me now, aren't you? I didn't deliver any of the talk.'

'No you didn't,' I said. 'But it would have been an educational failure if you *had* stuck to Plan A, and ploughed on with your talk. What I've just observed was a masterly example of clinical teaching. You had the flexibility to realise that something you weren't intending to discuss with the group (pain control) took priority over what you had initially planned. You picked up on the level of distress in the room and you made sure that everybody in the group could share their experience, if they wanted to. You took their concerns seriously, rather than brushing them on one side. And you gave them a clear account of what steps you were going to take next.'

Bernard looked relieved.

Our post-session feedback was wide-ranging. We talked about the transition from medical school to foundation, how to help juniors manage their feelings about the death of patients, the stresses of being a medical registrar and the relative lack of exposure to palliative care in the undergraduate curriculum.

'What would you like me to come and see next?' I asked.

'I teach undergraduate medical students,' Bernard said. 'Why don't you come and see an undergraduate teaching session in the hospice?'

*

A couple of weeks later I arrived at the hospice. As I walked through the door I was struck once again by the differences between hospitals and hospices; the soft colours on the walls, the artwork, the tea trolley doing its rounds for patients and their visitors – and above all, the absence of the frenetic rush that pervades so much of hospital practice. Why do we have to wait for the patients to be at the end of their lives before we provide this kinder environment?

But despite the fact that I had been so impressed by Bernard's previous session, I wasn't looking forward to the hospice observation. After Bernard had asked me to come and see him teach undergraduates, he had gone on to explain that in these sessions he used a 'goldfish bowl' technique with the twenty or so medical students forming a large circle around the edges of the room. He would sit in the middle of the circle with a day patient from the hospice. The students would then observe him as he had a conversation with the patient about their illness.

Familiar with the goldfish bowl technique from my training as a psychologist, I knew that it could provide the observers in the outer circle with a unique opportunity to see a conversation in the inner circle unfold in front of them. Yet at first the idea of putting terminally ill patients at the centre of the circle, with large numbers of medical students sitting around them and peering in, seemed grotesque. I felt there was something of the freak show about it, with the dying patient as the central exhibit.

With another consultant, I might have questioned this approach and encouraged them to consider a different way of teaching the medical students. But I had seen Bernard demonstrate an exceptional level of sensitivity to the junior doctors' needs. On the basis of the lunchtime session, I was willing to give him the benefit of the doubt.

In the event, my reservations couldn't have been more misplaced. Bernard had chosen his patients with enormous care. He knew the three patients well, and had treated each of them for many months. Barbara was in her forties, and dying of breast cancer; Shirley was twenty years older and had advanced ovarian cancer. The third patient, Edward, was in his seventies and had lung cancer. All three had been told by their doctors that any future treatment would be for symptom management rather than curing the disease. But whilst all three had terminal diagnoses, they were still living at home and attending the hospice as day patients.

Bernard interviewed them one at a time; an intense dialogue in the centre of the circle. Barbara spoke movingly about her fears of leaving her two sons without a mother. I noticed that many of the medical students in the outer circle had to wipe tears from their eyes. She also talked about insensitive doctors whom she had encountered at different points of her treatment, focusing on a particular cancer specialist who had been unable to understand her distress at the words *for advanced metastatic disease* printed on the outer packaging of some medication that she took at home. The consultant had said to Barbara, 'We've discussed your prognosis, and you know that the cancer is advanced. Why does it matter that this wording is printed on the box?'

Barbara described how this box of medication sat on her dressing table next to her favourite photo of her two sons, some earrings that belonged to her grandmother, and perfume given to her by her husband. Bernard understood that knowing and not-knowing could exist side by side. He appreciated that although on one level Barbara could have an intellectual understanding that her cancer was advanced, on another level she was distressed to have this fact thrown in her face every morning, when she sat at her dressing table. For Barbara the wording on the box served no clinical purpose, and instead intruded into the ordinary domestic pleasures of her family life – photos, earrings, perfume.

Shirley railed against her GP, who had failed to pick up the symptoms of ovarian cancer until the disease had already spread throughout her body. Despite repeated visits to the surgery, first she was reassured that she was suffering from irritable bowel syndrome. Later on, the GP suggested that perhaps she should be referred for counselling, because she seemed so anxious about her health. Turning round to address the medical students, Shirley said, 'If any of you become GPs, remember me. Don't fob off a middle-aged woman with a bloated stomach as having IBS. Listen to her and examine her thoroughly.'

There was a silence in the outer circle.

The final patient, Edward, had difficulty breathing, and he spoke quietly. The students in the outer circle craned forward to catch what he was saying.

'I smoked all my life, from the age of sixteen. We all did. I suppose you never think it's going to happen to you.'

Bernard nodded.

'I've had a good life,' Edward continued. 'I've been married nearly fifty years, three children and five grandchildren. I just want you doctors to do all you can to stop people smoking.'

Edward paused, with a rueful look on his face, then said, 'I wish somebody had tried harder to make me stop.'

In medical school lectures and seminars, I've often witnessed surprising levels of messing around; students playing with their mobile phones, passing notes and even surreptitious games of noughts and crosses. The students that morning in the hospice were among the most engaged that I have ever witnessed. I have little doubt that what they learned through observing the conversations in the centre of the goldfish bowl will stay with many of them throughout their working lives. And although my hospice visit took place over a decade earlier, subsequent research from the King's Fund highlighted how enabling students to hear patients speak about their personal experiences of care can be one of the most effective ways of enhancing their compassion.

I had also completely misjudged the impact on the patients of being asked to take part in the session. My fear was that there would be an element of voyeurism, and they would feel like a spectacle in the centre. I couldn't have been more wrong. What I hadn't adequately anticipated was the overwhelming desire that some patients have, to give something back to the doctors who treat them.

Bernard couldn't offer Barbara, Shirley or Edward a cure. But he could give each of them an opportunity to share their experiences with fledgling doctors who had their whole careers in front of them. In this way, the three of them clearly felt that after their deaths something constructive might come out of their individual suffering. Barbara needed oncologists to understand that patients don't want to be reminded of their prognosis as they go about their day-to-day business at home. Shirley felt passionately about the frequent misdiagnosis of the early symptoms of ovarian cancer. Edward hoped that more would be done to stop young people from smoking.

With each of these three patients, there was a change in their faces as their initial anxiety was transformed by the experience of being allowed to tell their stories. In fact there was a palpable sense, during the goldfish bowl session, that allowing these patients an opportunity to take part was tremendously healing.

*

I am not so naïve as to assume that all palliative care physicians are as compassionate as Bernard. Over the years, other clients have told me horrible tales of highly dysfunctional doctors working in hospices. Doctors whose kindness has been completely eroded by having to bear witness to death and dying every day.

But at its best, there is something about the specialty of palliative medicine that can lead to an exceptional form of patient care. Perhaps this is because palliative care physicians can't resort to a form of clinical omnipotence and hold out the promise of a cure to their patients. And whilst the medical aspects of the specialty – symptom management and pain control – are clearly vital, medicine alone will be insufficient if it isn't coupled with a capacity for engaging with the patient's suffering.

It's not easy to listen to patients' stories – to hear about the physical and psychological pain that they have experienced. Bernard didn't shy away from this task. And his capacity to respond empathically to others wasn't restricted to his patients but extended to those he encountered as a teacher. For whatever reason, Ellen was not open to Vartika's distress, whilst Bernard intuitively responded to the initial question raised by the junior doctor, and put his intended talk on one side.

The truth is that the best palliative care physicians have much to teach doctors in every other specialty.

3

Which Doctor

The minute Lola walked on to the ward she wanted to flee. This desire to get out of the hospital was so intense that she was unable to concentrate, or make any decisions, yet she knew that if she made a mistake, it could have hideous consequences. Every aspect of the ward – the people, the noises, the smells – felt unbearable. Three weeks into the job, the urgency with which she tried to escape the hospital resulted in her driving into another car in the staff car park. Three weeks after that, on her drive home, she crashed into a stationary car at a traffic light. Both accidents were her own fault. What was going on?

Lola was a doctor who had got through medical school and the early years of clinical practice without any difficulty whatsoever. Her life only started to unravel when she began her specialist training as an oncologist, treating cancer patients. After the second car crash she took a couple of days off work, and then, on her return, handed in her notice. 'I felt like a different person once I had resigned,' she told me.

She came to see me a couple of months later when the intense anxiety had subsided, but she was deeply confused about what to do next. Would she cope better if she became a GP and treated patients with a broader range of illnesses or should she abandon medicine entirely? And why hadn't she been able to cope with the oncology job for more than six weeks?

Quite early on in our first session, I asked Lola about her parents – what jobs had they done? Lola told me that her mother was a head teacher, and the 'driving force' of the family. Her father had been an engineer, a quiet, gentle man, who had died when Lola was ten. Lola's mother had found it hard to cope; on top of a demanding job she had to take care of four children on her own and she lapsed into depression. Most of Lola's close relatives lived in Hong Kong, but some cousins who lived in London helped out and eventually her mother was able to take responsibility for her family. The relationship between Lola and her mother, however, remained strained.

It wasn't difficult to guess what Lola's father had died of.

From the time of her father's death, Lola had set her heart on becoming a doctor. But the disruption to family life caused by her father's death took its toll, and she described herself as 'wild and disengaged' as a sixth-former, with little interest in her studies. Unsurprisingly, she didn't get the grades to go to medical school, so instead she studied biochemistry. Moving away from home felt like a liberation, and over the course of the three years she became increasingly focused on her academic work, eventually graduating with a first-class degree. At that point she reapplied to medical school, and was accepted.

In the first couple of years in the more traditional medical schools, students see only a few patients, but from the third year onwards, they spend more time on the wards. Lola described her experience in some of the different specialties; obstetrics was 'hanging around waiting for something to happen' whilst orthopaedics was 'a bit of a laugh'. And oncology?

Lola paused. And then she remembered that the first patient she had caught sight of in the oncology ward was a middle-aged Chinese man, bald from chemotherapy – just as she remembered her father had once looked. She had fainted at the foot of his bed. This was five years earlier, and she hadn't thought it significant at the time. Yet it was the only time that she had ever fainted in her entire medical school training.

Once Lola had qualified, she struggled with working out what she wanted to do with her career. She spent some time in A & E, then she went to New Zealand for a couple of years to work as a doctor. But she still wasn't sure. Meanwhile, her siblings were putting increasing pressure on her to return home to the UK, which, in the end, she did.

Back in the UK, she took a temporary locum post in oncology, which she found extremely distressing. I asked her what in particular she had found difficult, and she told me she had been shocked by how young some of the patients with cervical cancer were, and how poor the prognosis could be.

'The treatment was horrible,' she said, 'with all sorts of complications. I hated having to tell women that they wouldn't be able to have children.'

Yet despite the fact that she had struggled with her temporary post in oncology, Lola still went ahead and applied for a six-year specialty training programme, at the end of which (had she completed it) she could have been appointed as a consultant oncologist. Throughout the lengthy selection process for the oncology training scheme she was simultaneously applying for jobs outside medicine as a management consultant. Even when she got her oncology place she asked the management consultancy firm that had also offered her a job to keep it on hold for the next six months. From the beginning of her training in oncology, Lola was deeply unsure whether she had made the correct choice.

Lola had resigned from oncology before she first came to see me. She was aware that her intense distress during the six weeks she spent treating cancer patients was somehow linked to her father's death. And she described her relief when she made the decision not to continue in the specialty. 'I felt as if I was continually scratching open a wound,' was how she put it.

What was more puzzling was the way in which Lola had ignored all the earlier clues that she might find treating patients with cancer overwhelmingly difficult. She fainted just once in medical school – and that was at the sight of a patient receiving chemotherapy, who reminded her of her father. She'd tried out a locum post in oncology, and found it deeply upsetting. She crashed her car within weeks of starting her oncology training, in her rush to get out of the hospital. And still she continued – until she crashed her car for the second time, and realised that she couldn't go on.

Lola didn't come to see me for bereavement counselling (although I suggested that she might find it beneficial). We didn't focus on how she might have felt as a child when her father died. I don't know whether her emotional response as a ten-year-old was characterised by fury at being abandoned or guilt that she could have done more to help her parents, or by any other emotion. But what Lola's story shows is the overwhelming need that people have to make sense of their world through their work. Even though she eventually concluded that the task was too hard, part of her was powerfully drawn to helping patients who were suffering from the disease that killed her father.

In our early sessions, Lola toyed with the idea of leaving medicine entirely – in large part because she had been so traumatised by the six weeks she had spent on the oncology wards. But at the end of our sessions she realised that there were many aspects of medical work that she enjoyed, and that it was only being surrounded by patients with cancer that she couldn't manage. Lola decided to change direction, and successfully applied to train as a GP.

*

Tessa told me her mother had died, at the age of forty-one, when Tessa was eleven. She came from a family of four children, and she was the eldest. When we talked about her early family life, Tessa remembered that she had actually wanted to train as a doctor before her mother had become ill. Her grandfather had been a GP, and as a little girl, she had often stayed with her grandparents during the holidays and seen his patients walking up the garden path to the surgery next door to the house. But after her mother's death, her goal had switched from wanting to follow in her grandfather's footsteps and be a GP, to treating patients suffering from cancer.

'I put all of myself into my work,' Tessa said.

Whilst she won prizes and plaudits, this intense emotional investment in her work took its toll. In her late twenties she was diagnosed with Crohn's Disease – an autoimmune disorder of the gut. It's a horrible condition to manage as the symptoms include violent diarrhoea, difficulty absorbing food, severe pain and extreme fatigue. Although genetic predisposition and childhood infections are recognised as causing the condition, emotional stress influences the course that the disease takes.

For over twenty years Tessa had suffered from a particularly severe form of the disease, characterised by frequent hospital stays and different surgical interventions, interspersed with ever-decreasing periods of remission when she felt well. Tessa had tried reducing her hours and going part-time, but in the end realised that she had become too unwell to continue.

'I've had to give up work, in order to live,' was how she put it.

Tessa recognised that the intensity of her commitment to her patients made her ill. But why would a doctor continue working, for over a quarter of a century, when it extracted such a high personal cost? It's difficult to make sense of this without recourse to the psychoanalytic idea that people are driven, often without being aware, to seek ways in the present to deal with unresolved emotions from the past, especially from infancy and childhood.

John Ballatt and Penelope Campling describe this clearly:

> The unconscious motivation is often to heal a sick, or dead, family member and the guilt and fear of facing failure can become channelled into a relentless drive to work even harder. Unfortunately the choice of work brings not only the opportunity for reparation and healing but also repeats the experience of failing the incurable, which in turn, further feeds the associated emotional drive to apply oneself to this impossible task.

And that is exactly what happened to Tessa. She worked at this 'impossible task' until her own health failed.

Yet alongside the intensity of Tessa's commitment to patients with cancer, and her sorrow at having to take early retirement, was an enormous passion for life. When we discussed how she now wanted to make use of her medical knowledge and skills, she realised that she wanted to shift from illness to well-being. As an oncologist she had become interested in mindfulness meditation as a way of helping patients manage distressing and painful symptoms. Now she wanted to train as a mindfulness teacher and offer sessions to healthcare staff, as opposed to working directly with patients. And perhaps most important of all, in the absence of patients, for the first time in her life, she prioritised her own health over the health of others.

*

It's not difficult to see how the death of Lola's father and Tessa's mother influenced their specialty decisions. But parents aren't the only family members whose illness or death impact on a doctor's career choices. With other doctors, the experience of a sibling has been the critical factor.

I first became aware of this when observing a consultant give a lecture on asthma to a particularly disengaged group of medical students.

'You might think of asthma as a pretty trivial illness,' she began. 'With a few puffs on an inhaler there's nothing to worry about. But you would be wrong.'

She paused, to get the attention of the whole group.

'An asthma attack killed my twelve-year-old brother.'

This was twenty years ago. I've never forgotten it, and I suspect that many of those students present remember it as well. And what was this consultant's specialty? Respiratory medicine. The specialty that treats breathing difficulties. Including asthma.

I've also seen neurology trainees who have grown up with siblings suffering from multiple sclerosis and trainees specialising in the psychiatry of learning disability, who have learning-disabled siblings. The reparative urge isn't only induced by parental illness. And it isn't only caused by cancer. Illnesses occurring in any close family member can influence the career decisions that someone makes. Often the response (as with Lola, Tessa and the respiratory medicine consultant) is a desire to treat patients with the same disease that killed a beloved family member. Sometimes, however, as with Kevin, a doctor who switched from engineering to medicine after his sister died of leukaemia, it works a bit differently.

Kevin didn't want to train in haematology, the specialty that treats patients with leukaemia. Instead from the moment he started medical school, he only ever considered one specialty – obstetrics. When he came to see me he had completed medical school and had spent five years training in obstetrics. However, his career progression had ground to a halt because he couldn't pass his last specialty examination. This exam failure was puzzling because he consistently received excellent feedback from his supervisors for his clinical work and he had also completed a PhD in a leading academic research centre. Neither his clinical nor academic ability were in doubt. But he couldn't pass this one last exam.

What emerged from our sessions was that he had been drawn to obstetrics because he thought it would allow him to be surrounded by new life, rather than death. But of course if a doctor has chosen obstetrics for this reason, it is a doomed enterprise. Babies can be stillborn, or die shortly after birth. And very occasionally, mothers can die too. Whilst death and dying will be less of your daily diet at work if you are an obstetrician as opposed to an oncologist, you can't escape death entirely.

As we talked, it became clear that Kevin didn't really want to bear the responsibility of being a consultant obstetrician. He'd seen the drama that could ensue in obstetric emergencies, and he didn't want to be the person heading up the whole team. Yet this was the role he would be destined for, if he passed his final specialty examination. Kevin told me that he dreaded being held responsible for the death of a mother or a baby. Perhaps for him this responsibility felt unbearable because he knew, from his own family, what the death of a young person could feel like. I tentatively suggested to Kevin that perhaps his repeated examination failure was an unconscious solution to the problem of having to assume an intolerable burden of responsibility. As long as he kept on failing the exam, he could never become a consultant.

At the end of our sessions, Kevin reached the point where he felt able to leave clinical practice. Whilst previously he had attributed his repeated examination failure to stupidity or laziness, he came to see that perhaps it had served an important psychological function. He also decided that he would be happier working outside the hospital environment. Eventually he accepted a job with a pharmaceutical company, and he contacted me a few months later to tell me how much he was enjoying it. Although he missed seeing patients, his career change had brought him considerable psychological relief.

*

Every new service will have a first request for help – Client 001. Kelly was my first client in the service I set up in the autumn of 2008.

Just one month into her first job as an F1 doctor, Kelly walked into the office at the hospital education centre and announced that she wanted to quit. Her distress was so intense that the senior doctor in charge of foundation trainees did an assessment of suicide risk before she let Kelly leave her office and go home. A couple of days later, following an appointment with occupational health, Kelly went on an extended period of sick leave. It was also recommended that she should access support from the Careers Unit. Although she didn't know it, she became my Client 001.

In our first session Kelly was adamant that she would never return to medicine. Working as a doctor had made her physically sick – she vomited before she went into the hospital each day. Instead she wanted a non-medical job which involved working with children. A few weeks later she was able to see that perhaps she hadn't given clinical medicine much of a chance. After all, she had studied for five years to train as a doctor, and had then abandoned the career after working for less than five weeks. Although she was terrified at the prospect of going back to the hospital, maybe she would regret it if she jumped ship at this stage. Would she always ask herself whether medicine could have worked out?

A month or so after she had first walked out of her job, she remembered that at medical school she had enjoyed her placement with the community paediatrics team. What had fascinated her in particular was seeing how the paediatrician tried to understand the psychological causes of a child's behavioural problems. Perhaps she could work as a community paediatrician?

I didn't discount this idea when Kelly suggested it. In fact, I encouraged her to find out more about what the job entailed. But I also knew that you can't train as a community paediatrician without spending a number of years as an acute hospital-based paediatrician, including treating newborn babies. Given that she was terrified of carrying out technical procedures on adults (inserting a cannula, taking a blood sample), I wondered how she would manage to carry out the same tasks on tiny premature babies.

'What about child and adolescent psychiatry?' I asked.

Kelly had learnt nothing about this specialty in medical school. She agreed that it was worth exploring further, so I put her in touch with a consultant.

At our next session, Kelly told me she felt completely torn. Having spent some time in a child and adolescent psychiatry clinic, she agreed that she might enjoy the work. But this realisation was unwelcome. If she wanted to train in this specialty she would have to return to working as a foundation doctor – a prospect she found simply terrifying.

In our sessions it became increasingly clear that Kelly had a particular sensitivity to transitions. The move from primary to secondary school, from secondary school to sixth form college, from college to medical school and, most of all, from medical school to her first job, had all been problematic. This is not uncommon. And those individuals who have suffered repeated disappointments in life, or who have regularly had their confidence undermined, are more likely to experience difficulties at points of transition. Which is exactly what happened to Kelly.

Kelly found it helpful to see how her acute distress when she started her first job was a repetition of a long-standing pattern. With each of the earlier transitions she initially felt overwhelmed, but after a period of time she settled in and adjusted to her new school, college or university course. The fact that her first job had been in a town where she knew nobody had definitely contributed to her distress. Second time round, with some reluctance, she applied through the 'special circum-stances' route, citing her depression and anxiety. This allowed her to return to the hospital where she had completed her undergraduate training, and live amongst friends in a town where she had strong links.

The consultant in charge of the foundation trainees at this hospital was a particularly sensitive doctor whom I knew well. I was confident that Kelly was in good hands. But even with all the support in place, Kelly's anxiety remained problematic. When we spoke during the first two foundation placements, she wasn't sure if she would be able to get through the whole year.

A month into her third placement Kelly emailed me:

Thought I would just drop you a quick email to let you know how things are.

I have just started my psychiatry placement and am loving it so far. For the first time in medicine I feel I am finally enjoying something and I just wanted to thank you again for helping me to see that there is an area of medicine that I enjoy. Without your help I would have given up and never seen this.

End of story? Not exactly.

Perhaps predictably, Kelly suffered another mini-crisis when she moved into the second year of the foundation programme. She became acutely anxious about whether she was capable of fulfilling the additional responsibilities that doctors take on in the second year. She weathered that storm, but once she started applying for specialty training in psychiatry she worried whether she might end up having to move again. Either she stayed put, or changed her career – she wouldn't countenance a move. In the event, her application was successful and she started training as a psychiatrist, still based in the same town.

I contacted Kelly recently and asked permission to tell her story. She is married now and has two young children. Kelly told me that she is pleased that she stuck with her training, as she realises she has the potential to work as a consultant. But she also recognises that staying with it has come at a huge personal cost. The periods of intense anxiety linked to each job shift are shorter – but they haven't gone away.

When Kelly returns to work after her maternity leave she will be working part-time. This is something she wanted to do years before, but when she asked prior to having children, her request for part-time work on health grounds was denied. She wasn't regarded as sufficiently unwell.

'Why do you have to be at crisis point before there is any flexibility in the system?' she asked.

I didn't have a good answer. But I saw the irony in her question: doctors tell their patients that prevention is better than cure, yet a preventative ethos is frequently absent in medical training.

*

Kelly is not alone; personal experience of mental illness is known to be one of the reasons why a doctor might opt for a career in psychiatry. For example, a 2014 World Psychiatric Association (WPA) study across twenty-two countries found strong empirical evidence of the link between personal (and family) experience of mental illness and choosing to specialise in psychiatry. Of course it's not the only reason, and it doesn't apply in some blanket way to every psychiatrist. But if you compare a group of psychiatrists to a group of doctors who have chosen another specialty there is likely to be a higher incidence of personal or family mental health problems in the former group.

Dr Mike Shooter, former President of the Royal College of Psychiatrists, has talked openly about his own struggles with depression. In a remarkably candid interview, he described how his personal experience of mental illness – knowing what it feels like from the inside – has helped him care for his patients. Sometimes he tells patients how being depressed felt for him. He will then ask the patients if this was how they, too, experienced the illness. And in this way, a dialogue is opened up. His openness about his own periods of depression brings him closer to the patients and allows him to learn something valuable about them. Shooter is also aware that, when treating patients for an illness that one has suffered from oneself, there is always the danger of blurring one's own experience with that of the patient. But on balance, he feels that it has given him a particular understanding of the suffering endured by patients with a mental illness.

The notion that a doctor's capacity for healing stems from their own suffering – the so-called 'wounded healer' – has ancient roots. As an example, Plato's *Republic*, written in around 380 BC, contains the following verse:

> The most skilful physicians are those who, from their youth upwards, have combined with the knowledge of their art the greatest experience of disease . . . and should have had all manner of diseases in their own person.

*

In contemporary psychotherapeutic practice this idea of the 'wounded healer' is closely associated with the writings of Carl Jung who suggested that through the experience of personal suffering, the healer can acquire a deep wisdom which they can then use for the benefit of their patients. But Jung was also aware that there was always the potential that such healers could over-identify with patients, feeling their pain too deeply, reawakening wounds of their own.

Over the years I have seen many trainees whose personal experience of mental illness has attracted them to psychiatry – and whose commitment and empathy have been enhanced in the ways that Shooter has described. Sadly, as we'll see in a later chapter, I have also encountered doctors whose progression through psychiatry training has been derailed by severe and recurrent episodes of mental illness. It doesn't always work out for the best.

*

It's not only with psychiatrists that there is a clear link between personal experience of mental illness and wanting to help others who suffer from similar conditions. This link applies to psychologists and psychotherapists as well. And it applies to me.

My older brother is autistic. As a child I can remember times when he was extremely agitated and distressed. When I was six, my mother suffered from a serious episode of depression following the death of her beloved sister from cancer. As a teenager at boarding school, I became so unwell with depression that I had to come home for half a term while I received outpatient psychiatric treatment. And as an adult I have experienced further episodes of depression following a traumatic bereavement and also after the birth of two of my children.

I am in no doubt that my personal and family experiences of psychological distress played a part in my decision to train as a psychologist. If one has never witnessed psychological problems close-up, or experienced them oneself, it is harder (although not impossible) to become interested in what goes on in other people's minds. These personal or family experiences teach you – often from a young age – that minds matter. But it's not always easy to talk openly about the ways in which one's own mental health difficulties have affected one's career. Amongst doctors, there's tremendous stigma attached to any admission of psychological problems (which makes Mike Shooter's openness all the more extraordinary). Given that studies have repeatedly demonstrated that medical students and junior doctors see psychiatry as being unlike all the other specialties, it's almost as if the stigma spreads beyond the individual to infect the profession of psychiatry as a whole.

*

Lola, Tessa, Kevin and Kelly. Four individuals whose career stories show how the threads of family life ripple through the decisions that people make about their work. But these few stories don't convey the sheer number of specialty choices facing each doctor. Of course young people qualifying in other professions such as law or accountancy face choices – but not on the same scale as doctors. So how many specialties re there?

It's a simple question that doesn't have an equally simple answer.

The division of medical knowledge and tasks into specialties and sub-specialties doesn't map on to a physical reality. In chemistry, for example, an element is defined on the basis of its atomic structure, so a carbon atom remains a carbon atom wherever one is in the world and occupies the same place in the Periodic Table of Elements. In terms of medical specialties, however, different countries carve up the medical universe in many different ways. So in the UK doctors have to choose between sixty-six specialties, which in turn branch out further into thirty-two sub-specialties. In the USA there are thirty-seven specialties, which then branch out into eighty-six sub-specialties whilst in Australia there are eighty-five specialties with no further sub-specialisation. Yet one thing that unites all of these countries is that in the second decade of the twenty-first century, doctors have to navigate their way through an enormous array of options. And some doctors make choices that they later come to regret.

A consistent finding in studies is that a significant minority of doctors feel they have chosen the wrong specialty. For example, a 2013 survey of over 7,000 doctors in the States reported that between a third and a quarter were not happy with the specialties that they had chosen. Specialty dissatisfaction was particularly acute amongst mid-career doctors. Other studies have looked within particular specialties, and similar patterns emerge; nearly 20% of oncology and surgical trainees in the States wouldn't choose their specialty again. A whopping 34% of obstetric trainees, in an admittedly small study in the UK, regretted their specialty choice. An exception to the rule was anaesthetists, where a recent American study found that over 94% were satisfied that they had chosen the right career. Unfortunately such high satisfaction bucks the general trend.

It is clear that many doctors are disappointed with their specialty decisions. This doesn't only represent a widespread degree of personal dissatisfaction in the medical profession; it also has ramifications for patients. Not surprisingly, when doctors are dissatisfied at work, they tend to have more dissatisfied patients. And the patients of more dissatisfied doctors are less likely to stick to the treatment plans that they have been prescribed. Dissatisfaction is contagious.

So what do we know about the process of specialty decision making? And how can we use this knowledge to help doctors make better decisions?

There's no shortage of studies that have asked doctors why they chose their particular specialty. From the 1950s onwards, thousands of papers in medical journals have looked at every conceivable specialty, including reports from far-flung corners of the globe. Some researchers have suggested that specialty choice boils down to personality and there's a micro-industry of studies that have examined whether surgeons are a particular breed with a distinct 'surgical' personality. As an example, over forty years ago a group of Harvard researchers compared the personalities of medical and surgical trainees using the Rorschach inkblot test. With this method subjects are presented with pictures of inkblots; the number of responses and the nature of each response are recorded and later analysed.

Rorschach is a controversial method, and one can imagine that the subjects (all young Harvard doctors) might have been somewhat sceptical at having their personalities assessed in this way.

The aim of the study was to explore whether the surgeons were more 'aggressive, rigid, insensitive, impersonal, hostile, extroverted, explosive and possibly more energetic and ambitious'. And the conclusion?

> The common stereotype of the cold, aloof, and aggressive surgeon was not confirmed.

It might be tempting to dismiss this conclusion on the basis that the Rorschach test is nothing more than pseudoscience. However, there is a resurgence of interest in Rorschach and a recent review in a leading psychological journal concluded that the method is reliable. Also, there are other studies using standardised personality questionnaires that agree with the Harvard findings. Yet again, there are studies that disagree, which have concluded that surgeons are indeed more extravert than doctors in other specialties, as well as being less warm and considerate to others. In terms of there being a distinct surgical personality the jury is still out. But after half a century of research there is little compelling evidence of a simple link between personality and the decision to opt for a particular specialty.

Three findings, however, occur with such frequency in different specialties, and across countries and continents, tha they would be hard to dispute. And whilst it is my job, rat than my clients', to read up on the academic literature specialty choice, these three issues are ones that doctors talk to me about, without any prompting, in sessions.

*

'So what were the reasons you decided to train as a GP?' I asked Zac.

After a moment's pause, Zac launched into a long and detailed response:

'I was inspired by the senior partner in the practice where I worked as a foundation trainee. She was a very good doctor; a sound knowledge base, and committed to a certain vision of general practice. Ethical – to her core. A key player locally. Quite eminent. Yet canny and streetwise. Plus she looked after all the doctors in the team.'

Zac didn't know it, but he'd given me a textbook description of the most common reason why junior doctors choose a particular specialty. Role models.

In the course of an individual's medical school and post-graduate training they will encounter hundreds of qualified doctors – in lectures, seminars, consulting rooms, ward rounds and in operating theatres. When asked why they chose a particular specialty, junior doctors will almost inevitably refer back to one or two role models they hold in high esteem. It's the enthusiasm, commitment, knowledge and expertise of more senior doctors that draws juniors into a particular specialty.

Sadly, the opposite is true as well. When medical students or junior doctors encounter cynical, ill-informed, callous seniors, it corrodes enthusiasm that they might otherwise have felt for a particular specialty. This also happened to Zac. Alongside general practice, he'd considered specialising in palliative medicine. But he'd been put off by one of the senior doctors in the local hospice.

'She was pedantic, and sour,' Zac told me. 'Stuck on detail, sarcastic and game playing. I decided I didn't want to end up like her.'

Perhaps if Zac had encountered a palliative care physician like Bernard he might have made a different career choice.

Zac's experience was echoed in the title of an academic medical education paper on role models: 'Trying on Possible Selves'. Juniors like Zac look to their seniors for representations of the sort of doctor that they aspire to be in future.

*

The second influence on specialty choice relates to the issue of role models – prior experience of that particular specialty. Medical students and junior doctors tend to choose specialties that they have enjoyed in medical school and in the early years of clinical practice. In many ways this is a sensible approach to career decision making, and Lola's experience (where she ignored the fact that she found her temporary post in oncology extremely distressing) shows that it is wise for doctors to think carefully about their prior experience of a specialty before opting for it in the longer term.

But prior experience is never a perfect test. One might have been unlucky in the particular department that one was assigned to, and gained a highly skewed sense of what working in the specialty would be like. For example, one doctor who came to see me had initially discounted psychiatry because during her medical school psychiatry placement she had felt inadequately supported on a forensic ward with violent male offenders. The experience had frightened her. But in our sessions she came to see that the placement was probably an unsuitable one for a medical student so it would be a mistake to rule out all psychiatric specialties on the basis of this one experience. She eventually chose to specialise in old-age psychiatry.

Another obvious problem with using prior experience to guide one's specialty choice is that given the huge number of specialties and sub-specialties, there are many that a medical student or junior doctor will never routinely encounter; they may not even know that these specialties exist. In the States, medical students use the elective period during the fourth year to choose their specialty, and they have space in the timetable to choose. In the UK the elective period and specialty choice are not linked in the same way, as specialty decisions are made a few years later down the line. The whole process of finding out about some of the smaller niche specialties that aren't routinely covered in medical school is often left to chance.

Occasionally with doctors I've felt a bit like a matchmaker; I've suggested an alternative option to somebody who didn't even know that the specialty existed and they go on to fall in love with this new line of work. This happened with Kate, a paediatric trainee who suffered from recurrent severe depression. Like many paediatric trainees who were having doubts about the specialty, it was the acute aspects of paediatrics, and particularly seriously ill newborn babies, that she found hardest to manage. I was unsure whether Kate would ever enjoy the demands of acute hospital paediatrics and I also thought she might struggle with the child protection aspects of working in the community; a doctor needs to be particularly resilient if their work regularly includes assessing children who have been abused.

At secondary school Kate had seriously considered applying for speech and language therapy, a non-medical career. However, as it was clear that she was going to get excellent grades in all her subjects, her teachers persuaded her that she should instead apply for medicine. Throughout her years at medical school she had volunteered to teach refugees spoken English at a local community centre, and she had enjoyed this work enormously. Kate was gentle and empathic with exceptional communication skills. Despite feeling overwhelmed by looking after acutely sick children, she always got excellent feedback from her patients and their parents.

Building on Kate's long-term interest in language, and the fact that she was a doctor with the sensitivity to discuss life-changing news with parents – such as the fact that their baby was profoundly deaf – I suggested to her that she might like to explore audio-vestibular medicine. This is a specialty in which doctors treat patients with disorders of hearing and balance. It's outpatient-based work, in which doctors rarely have to confront an acute clinical emergency. But it requires patience and attention to detail, together with an empathic capacity to imagine the psychological isolation that deafness can cause. Kate took up my suggestion.

Different specialties make widely differing psychological demands on the practitioner. As a psychologist I have found it profoundly rewarding when I have helped doctors like Kate who were failing in one specialty to identify an alternative in which they can thrive. Kate has now almost completed her specialty training in audio-vestibular medicine and, although she remains vulnerable to depression, moving away from acute paediatrics has transformed her working life.

*

The first two issues – the role models that a doctor encounters and their prior experience of a particular specialty – have always had an important impact on specialty decisions. We learn about the world and make decisions based on our experience, so how could it be otherwise? There's evidence, however, that a third factor has grown in importance in recent years, and also that, whereas formerly it was much more of a concern to women, it is now important to doctors of both sexes. What is it?

Work–life balance.

Newly qualified doctors today are less willing to devote their entire lives to their patients, at the expense of their own families, than their predecessors were. The issue of work–life balance has a much more significant impact on the specialties that doctors choose to follow, than it did in the past. So for example a 2015 study from researchers in Oxford concluded:

Domestic circumstances were a much more important consideration when choosing a specialty for the graduates of 2008–2012 compared with those of 1999–2002. Across the cohorts, female doctors rated domestic circumstances as having greater importance than male doctors, but its sharp increase in importance over the years was observed in both men and women.

This finding is not limited to the UK. A similar shift has been reported in the USA, with the Director of Medical Education at the Association of American Medical Colleges observing that 'The millennials seem to be more inclined than previous generations of physicians to trade some of their income for more control of their hours.'

Studies in Australia and Canada have reached the same conclusion.

What this means in practice is that factors such as the length of postgraduate training, the possibility of minimising evening or weekend commitments and the position of part-timers are ones that many contemporary junior doctors agonise over when choosing their specialty.

*

In essence, choosing one's specialty is a complex psychological decision. It's not surprising therefore that these three major factors – role models, prior experience and work–life balance – are mentioned in studies throughout the world. Why would a doctor in Birmingham, Alabama be less influenced by having a positive experience of a particular specialty in training than a doctor in Birmingham, England? And why would doctors in one country want to spend less time with their family than doctors in another? Many influence transcend national boundaries.

Other influences don't travel across the globe in the same way. A 2015 study of over 15,000 doctors in the UK reported that student debt had influenced the specialty choice of 2.8% of male doctors and 2.1% of female doctors. Concerns about paying back one's debt therefore don't appear to be a major factor in the UK – yet. This study followed up doctors who had graduated from UK medical school between 2008 and 2012. This means that all of the doctors in this study had left medical school before 2012 when the threefold tuition fee increase came into effect. The earliest that this increase might be detected in specialty choice decisions would be in doctors who graduate from four-year postgraduate courses in 2016 and choose their specialties in the December of the following year. Time will tell.

In the US in 2012, the median indebtedness at graduation for medical students was $170,000, and more than a quarter of students graduate with debts of over $200,000. Not surprisingly, these huge debts have a significant impact on specialty choice decisions. Despite going into medical school with all sorts of altruistic aspirations, financial reality kicks in, and students are forced to make some tough choices. A 2014 study in the US found that students with higher debt were more likely to choose a specialty with higher average annual income, were less likely to plan to practise in poor, under-served locations, and were less likely to choose primary care. Even more concerning is that increasing financial debt has been shown to correlate with residents' self-reports of increasing depression, and even suicidal ideation.

Historically in the UK, with state-funded university education and the majority of doctors working in the NHS, money wasn't a major factor in specialty choice. But as with many things, sooner or later much of what happens in the US finds its way across the Atlantic. The influence of student debt on specialty choice in the US may well be a portent of things to come, as the longer-term impact of increased student debt works its way through the system.

*

Doctors don't only face the challenge of choosing the right specialty. They also have to make the right decision at the right time. With some doctors, like Neil, the issue of timing has been central to their difficulties.

On the face of it, Neil's story was straightforward. He was at the point in his second foundation year when doctors are expected to choose their specialty, and he had decided to apply for the lab-based specialty of pathology. It takes at least five years for a doctor to progress from junior pathologist to the stage where they are eligible to be appointed as a consultant. This ordered progression through the ranks is achieved by gaining a place on a specialty training scheme.

Neil emailed me asking for help because he had an interview the following week for the pathology training scheme and he was feeling nervous. A particular focus of his anxiety was that, eighteen months earlier, he had had some time out due to depression. Now he was worried that the gaps in his CV would result in him being marked down at the interview.

As there were only a few days before the interview, I immediately got back to Neil and offered him an appointment. In our email exchange Neil expressed his gratitude for my prompt response. On the day itself, however, he was about fifteen minutes late. Pressed for time, because we now had just forty-five minutes rather than the normal sixty, I cracked on with the stated task of helping him prepare for the interview. We didn't manage to finish by the end of the session, so Neil asked if we might schedule a further meeting at the beginning of the following week. While he was still in the meeting room I phoned a colleague, rearranged my diary and squeezed him in.

When Neil arrived twenty-five minutes late for our second appointment, I was irritated, not least because I had reorganised my day to fit him in. With some effort I managed to park my irritation, and started to think about the psychological meaning of his lateness.

'I wonder if your lateness is your way of communicating to me that you don't want to go to the pathology interview this week?' I commented.

An immediate look of relief spread across Neil's face. He began to tell me that he didn't feel ready to commit himself to one specialty and wished he could get a bit more clinical experience before he made a final decision. What he really wanted to do was to stop the clock, and withdraw from the application process. For my part, I felt as if he had unconsciously been trying to get me to understand these doubts by turning up late to the first session, but I had been swept up by the practical task of helping him prepare for the interview. So he then had to be *really, really* late in order to get through to this dense psychologist – and luckily, the second time around, I got the message.

Sometimes, with clients, you will have a few sessions and then never hear what happens in the longer term. But on other occasions doctors will keep in touch, and tell you the next chapter of their story. This is what happened with Neil. Once it had become clear that he wanted to withdraw from the interview process, we agreed to broaden the focus beyond interview preparation, and scheduled some additional sessions to review his future career choices. At the end of these sessions Neil decided that he was indeed still committed to pathology, but he wanted to have a bit more experience in general medicine before he headed off to the lab. He also wanted to spend three months travelling, as a much-needed break, before he embarked on his five-year pathology training.

So that is what he did. And he kept in contact, emailing me about a year later to say that this time he had successfully gone through the interview process and was looking forward to starting his training as a pathologist.

Neil struggled to articulate (or even to know) what he wanted in his working life. He needed an extra year after foundation to make up his mind. In the past this would have been unremarkable, as it was common for junior doctors to do short-term jobs in different specialties, for a number of years, before they made their final specialty decisions. Previous experience of the specialty, although not perfect, is probably the most reliable way of finding out whether one is suited to that line of work. Nowadays medical training across the world has become packaged into a one-size-fits-all system predicated on the notion that all doctors take the same amount of time to progress through the different stages. We know that other developmental milestones (growth, sexual maturity, finding a long-term partner) don't happen according to a rigid timetable. Not everyone gets married at the age of thirty-one. But in both the UK and the US there are set points in medical training when people are expected to choose their specialty. The idea of taking extra time over this decision is often poorly received. And trainees are frightened to ask.

At least in the UK, however, junior doctors seem to be forcing the system to allow them more time. When the new system of training was introduced in 2005, the expectation was that all juniors would progress straight from foundation into their specialty training. But as we will see later, year on year, more trainees opt to take an extra year before they pin their colours to the mast and continue with their specialty training. This is good news if it increases the probability that doctors will end up in a specialty that suits them.

*

It's not surprising that some doctors need more time before they are ready to commit to one specialty. A sound choice can require a doctor to take so many different factors into account: previous experience of different specialties; length of training; money; finding an option that will fit in with family demands; minimising aspects of medical work that one has previously found particularly stressful; personal and family illness; bereavements. And of course this is not a complete list – merely some of the most common issues that doctors have talked to me about over the years.

But an appreciation of the psychological richness of the task hasn't permeated medical training. Despite all the studies showing that significant numbers of doctors regret their specialty choice, many consultants see the whole process as unproblematic. So sometimes, when running training workshops for senior clinicians on how best to support their trainees, my psychological approach has been rejected outright.

On one memorable occasion, a consultant obstetrician sitting in the back row of the seminar room raised his hand and said, 'I would be mortified if one of my trainees came to talk to you about their career. It would be a failure on my part, because I can't see what they could learn from you that I wouldn't be able to teach them.'

'Humility?' I suggested.

(Actually I didn't say that – it only came to me as I was biking home. In the moment I was so outraged that my jaw clamped shut and I said nothing.) This particular consultant's question was predicated on a simplistic notion of how one helps somebody to reach a robust decision. Undoubtedly he would have known much more about the comparative prestige of different training schemes, or how best to build one's CV. But would he have cared about anything else? Specialty decisions are sedimentary: layer upon layer of personal and family influences, the chance factors of who one encounters, the role models who inspire one or turn one away from a specialty for life. And as with rock formation, these layers build up over a long period of time.

So how *can* we help the next generation of doctors make better choices so that they don't have to come banging on my door for help?

I'm not advocating long-term psychotherapy or Rorschach inkblot tests, or even in-depth career counselling. Some doctors need specialist psychological support in the task of specialty choice, but the majority don't.

However, *all* doctors need to approach the task with their eyes wide open. They need to remain curious both about themselves and about the full range of available options. This will only happen if the whole issue of specialty choice is reframed. Starting from the beginning of medical school and continuing throughout training, there must be ongoing discussion about specialty choice in particular, and the emotional demands of medicine in general.

A student doesn't enter medical school as a *tabula rasa*. All students should be taught that things that have happened in their life before medical school (pressure to follow in parental footsteps, family or personal illness, divorce) might have an impact on how they experience different specialties. Both students and qualified doctors should be encouraged to be alert to atypical responses (fainting/crashing cars/unexplained exam failure) – not in order to reach quick, simplistic conclusions but just to start wondering whether these are vital clues to aspects of work that might be overwhelming. They need to think carefully about the patients they enjoy treating – the clinical puzzles they love to solve, as well as those tasks that they find too traumatic. Or perhaps just not very interesting.

I am advocating this 'eyes wide open' approach because of the countless stories of mistaken career choices that doctors have recounted over the last ten years. Yet it's also an approach that is entirely congruent with contemporary models of occupational psychology. A leading psychologist in the States, Tom Kreishok, argues that, although a conscious, rational approach to career decision making has a role to play, rationality has its limits. He suggests that if we *really* want to help people make better career decisions we need to encourage them to think about, and inhabit, the feelings associated with their day-to-day experiences at work.

If this simple message had been reinforced throughout the years of medical training, Lola, and many other doctors, might have been able to choose more wisely.

4

Brief Encounter

_____

The initial email was short and to the point, requesting an appointment as soon as possible. There were no further details bar a name, Peter, and the fact that he would be travelling for a considerable distance to get to me. I responded suggesting some dates, and a time was arranged with minimum delay or fuss.

On the appointed day, I opened the door to a tall, good-looking man of African heritage whose face seemed creased with worry. Once in my office, he paused before sitting down, as if he was uncertain whether he wanted to stay or go. Eventually we both sat down, and I waited.

Without prompting, Peter began telling me his story. He had grown up in London although both his parents had been born in West Africa. He'd attended medical school in the north of England but had moved back south to complete his postgraduate training. Now thirty-five years old, he had been working as an obstetrician in London for the past two years.

He was eligible to apply for consultant posts, but he was having doubts. Did he really want to be delivering babies for the next thirty years?

Recently his dilemma had become more pressing as a consultant obstetrician post had come up in the hospital where he was currently working, and everybody there was keen for him to apply. That the application deadline was only two weeks away was the main reason why he wanted to meet with me. He just wasn't sure whether he wanted the job.

'I'm quite an anxious person,' he told me, 'and I struggle with the acuteness of the labour ward.'

'Is this new?' I asked.

'No – it's always been like that. I kept on hoping that things would change. But I've completed my training and nothing has shifted.

'I'm quite introverted,' he added, 'and I don't really like being in charge of a large team in the labour ward – the anaesthetists, midwives and nurses. I prefer one-on-one. It's an effort being on call and having to take charge in an emergency. And it will only get worse when I'm a consultant.'

As an alternative, Peter explained, he was seriously considering changing track and applying to train as a GP. In fact he had applied for GP training on four separate occasions during his obstetrics training. Each time he was accepted and each time he turned the offer down, and continued in obstetrics. Yet he continued in the specialty, despite the fact that he invariably found the labour ward an emotional struggle.

'I want a better work–life balance in future,' Peter told me. Then there was a pause. 'I keep my private life quite separate from work – but I don't want to be overwhelmed by my work so I have no energy for a private life, when I get home.'

There was another, longer pause.

'There's also an issue of my sexual orientation. I'm gay. A couple of people at work know, but most don't. And neither do my family.'

I thought back to some of the homophobic jibes I had heard over the years: the not so subtle innuendo about a distinguished physician who was a 'confirmed bachelor' or the raised eyebrows in the outpatient clinic when a gay patient left the consulting room. And studies that have looked at sexual attitudes within the medical profession paint a disquieting picture. For example, a study published in 2015 by researchers at Stanford University in California found that over a quarter of medical students in the US and Canada who identified themselves as belonging to a minority sexual orientation concealed this at medical school. So Peter was not alone in feeling the need to remain in the closet. Medicine, it would appear, is not the easiest profession in which to be openly gay.

Peter continued his tale. Each time he had applied for GP training he'd felt relief at the prospect of removing himself from the demands of the labour ward. But his family and friends thought it would be a waste of all the time he had spent in obstetrics if he changed course. The nearer he got to completing his training the more he wanted to leave, and the more everyone around him argued that he should stay. Now, the need to decide whether or not to apply for the consultant post in his current trust had galvanised his thinking.

'Last week, when I emailed you, I was really unsure, but I spent the weekend thinking things through, and my gut feeling is not to apply. The job has got a heavy clinical load in labour ward with little time for anything else, and I just don't want it.'

I had a sense that Peter had made his decision and that he might not actually need any further sessions. 'It's fine, if you get home and decide that you don't want any more sessions with me,' I told him. 'Sometimes preparing for a session like the one today can be enough – and people realise they don't need to delve any deeper into their career.'

Thanking me for my time, Peter then left with a firm hand-shake.

That afternoon, my mind turned back to our meeting: the urgent request to see me, and travelling halfway across the country for the session even though he had already made up his mind not to apply for the job; the large body in the too-small chair, almost as if he had outgrown something that he had been sitting on; applying to train as a GP on four occasions, but never being able to make the switch; continuing for eight years in a specialty which he had never really enjoyed.

I started to wonder how his sexual orientation might have impacted on his choice of specialty. Two decades ago a young man growing up in his community, where being openly gay probably felt impossible, might well have struggled with the feelings he experienced when he examined some of his male patients. I don't for a second think that he ever behaved inap-propriately – and he might not have been conscious of the source of his discomfort – but perhaps he wanted to minimise contact with male patients. Could he have been drawn to obstet-rics, even though he knew that he found the labour ward extremely stressful, because it was the one specialty where he knew all his patients would be women?

This is an issue that applies to all doctors, whether straight, gay, or whatever. All doctors have to be sufficiently at ease with the desires that a particular patient may evoke in them, so that they recognise the attraction while resisting the temptation to respond. Equally, it is unhelpful if the recognition of an attraction to a patient results in an overwhelming self-persecutory response.

Working on the labour ward, you can never escape the risk of a woman experiencing a massive haemorrhage. This is a clinical emergency which can rapidly escalate into a clinical catastrophe – with the added complication that one has to consider the safety of both mother and child. As somebody who hated acute clinical emergencies, Peter would be better suited to the GP consulting room. I wondered whether it had taken Peter a long time to be sufficiently comfortable with his own sexuality, so that the thought of treating male patients no longer felt problematic. And perhaps coming to see me and being able to tell me that he was gay – even though he still kept his sexuality secret from his family and most people at work – was one of the final pieces of the jigsaw? I obviously thought that his sexuality had no bearing on his choice of specialty, and could see no problem at all with him training to be a GP.

Mulling all of this over, my prediction was that he wouldn't need to come and see me again.

And he never did.

*

Although I only saw Peter once, he made me curious. How well does medical training equip young people to carry out intimate examinations of another person's body? After all, some of the students may never have seen the genitals of a person of the opposite sex – let alone touched them.

My colleague Helena came to mind. She was an older obstetrician coming up to retirement – somebody who held a senior training role in the specialty and had supervised generations of medical students and junior doctors. Helena is also a friendly and open-minded individual, with whom it is easy to discuss sexual and emotional matters. I emailed her, asking how she helps neophyte doctors manage their feelings about carrying out intimate examinations, and how she approaches the possibility with them that an erotic dimension could enter into the process. This was her reply:

> This is an issue which has never come up and has certainly never been discussed in any training forum. This is not to say that it could never be an issue, but we never discuss even the possibility and how to handle it. We perhaps disassociate the clinical aspects of the patient assessment from any emotional process.

I was astounded by her response. As a psychologist, I don't examine any body parts. And I don't touch, beyond an occasional handshake at a first or last meeting. I listen, I talk (and of course I look out for non-verbal signals such as blushing, shifting around in the chair or avoiding my gaze). The verbal currency that forms the basis of my professional exchange is qualitatively different from that of the doctor who is shown and touches parts of the body hidden from everyday view. Yet an essential part of my training as a psychologist was to make me aware of the emotional dynamics embedded in any verbal exchange with a client.

I am alert to the power of the 'transference' that clients bring to any encounter. This is the notion, originating in Freud's work, that people unconsciously displace on to the therapist feelings or thoughts derived from earlier key relationships in their life. In other words, a client may respond to me *as if* I were their father, or their mother, or some other key person in their life. This is an everyday occurrence in my work with clients:

Natalie, a GP trainee, tells me about a recent incident at work. Her surgery was running late and she knew that patients were stacking up in the waiting room. In a rush to get through a particular consultation, she unthinkingly pressed a key on the computer and brought up the notes of the patient who was next in the queue, rather than the patient who was actually sitting in front of her. When it then came to issuing a prescription, she issued it for the wrong patient. Although she realised her mistake before the patient left the room, it had left her with considerable anxiety.

After Natalie has finished describing the incident, I am left wondering which part of the story to pick up. Should I ask whether there was something about this particular patient that might have distracted her, or perhaps I should hone in on her anxiety? There is a pause as I ponder which avenue it might be most helpful to explore.

Natalie interrupts my thinking:

'You probably think I'm too stupid to be a doctor. That's what my dad always said.'

Natalie experienced my pause '*as if*' it was laden with something.

But transference isn't a one-way street. Responding '*as if*' one person was somebody else doesn't just happen to clients. A comparable process happens to the practitioner, and is known in the trade as 'counter-transference'. Again this is a ubiquitous feature of psychological work:

Following a session with a desperately unhappy medical student, Frances, I am left with overwhelming feelings of anxiety. In part this is due to her previous history of self-harm, and her isolation, but I find myself entertaining the fantasy (which I obviously don't voice) that perhaps she should come and live with me for a while, until she feels better able to care for herself. Even though I see many clients in comparable states of distress, and can usually manage my anxiety on my own, I have an urgent need to discuss my concerns with my clinical supervisor. I telephone her as soon as Frances has left and in this discussion I become aware that Frances is the same age as my daughter. There was something about Frances's vulnerability that momentarily made me feel an intense desire to scoop her up and become her mother – hence the unspoken fantasy of offering her a home. Counter-transference.

A couple of weeks later I met up with two colleagues who were also involved with supporting Frances. It emerged that they had both been left feeling unusually anxious. But these other colleagues didn't have daughters of the same age as Frances – so they weren't wanting to look after her because in some way she reminded them of their daughters. There was also something going on with Frances that made those supporting her hyper-aware of her extreme vulnerability. Later still, Frances told me that she had been abused by her stepfather as a child.

In other words, my counter-transference to each client is partly a product of my personal history (Frances reminded me of my daughter) but also due to the unique history of the client, (Frances had been abused and unconsciously managed to project feelings of overwhelming anxiety into those who were tasked with providing her support).

Transference and counter-transference are the warp and weft of psychological work. A key part of our training is learning how to step back and discern patterns in how the client unconsciously responds to you (transference) and how you unconsciously respond to the client (counter-transference). But these processes are not confined to the consulting room. They are ubiquitous phenomena that happen all the time, in our interactions with others.

Back when I was a secondary school teacher, I can remember pupils putting up their hand and saying 'Mum' instead of 'Ms Elton'. For a second they had unconsciously responded to me as if I was their mother. Typically they were then incredibly embarrassed. And it's not just children. At work, some of the spats we get into (and our alliances) may have their roots in our relationships with siblings. And how we respond to authority often harks back to our early relationships with our parents. Transference and counter-transference happen between doctors and patients, therapists and clients, teachers and students, priests and parishioners, bosses and junior staff. They are everywhere. What's different about being a psychologist is that not only are we taught about it, but we are also allowed (and even expected, in some theoretical circles) to talk about it. With the exception of psychiatrists, and GPs, doctors are rarely afforded this luxury.

Yet even for psychologists there are times when discussions about transference and counter-transference get tricky, and that's when one starts to stray into the territory of sex. The client may experience you as hyper-critical (as Natalie did), or uninterested, chaotic, preoccupied – *any* emotional state, depending upon their own developmental history. So erotic feelings towards the psychologist can definitely be part of the rich mix. And the same is true for the psychologist, where an erotic dimension can enter into the counter-transference.

My sessions with doctors focus on helping them think in depth about their work. Whilst all sorts of emotions can emerge in the consulting room, typically the discussions don't become erotically charged. But in my training as a counselling psychologist I have worked with clients who were struggling with different sexual issues. I know what it feels like when you find yourself positioned as the object of desire (or the object of sexualised hatred) within a therapeutic relationship. And if I hark back to an even earlier stage of my career, when I was in my early twenties, I can remember noting a certain A-level student who seemed particularly keen to hang around after lessons and talk to me. There was definitely a sexual frisson in the air; I never transgressed any professional boundary, but there was a small part of me that felt quite flattered.

*

Erotic potential is never that far from the surface. Yet the response of my senior obstetrics colleague when I asked how she prepares medical students to carry out intimate examinations suggests that a defensive shield has been placed around the medical profession as a whole. The received wisdom seems to be that sexual stuff infiltrates other professions, but doctors are immune. Despite a vast literature on whether it is better to use manikins, anaesthetised patients or volunteer teaching associates to train students in carrying out gynaecological examinations, there was almost nothing written about helping students manage their sexual feelings. Just like intimate body parts, this topic was hidden from view.

In 1997, Terri Kapsalis, an American cultural critic and health educator, wrote the wonderfully titled *Public Privates* – a detailed study of how doctors are taught gynaecology. In the book Kapsalis commented how within the canon of medical education, journal articles typically fail to discuss 'the precarious relationship between pelvic exams and sex acts'. This supposed desexualisation becomes untenable when one learns that in the early 1970s a number of medical schools in the USA hired prostitutes as 'patient simulators' for their medical students to practise on. In choosing prostitutes, Kapsalis argues, medical educators inadvertently situated the pelvic examination as an act with sexual connotations.

Medical students are far from stupid, and of course they discussed the sexual potential of intimate examinations. But these discussions took place in private conversations, rather than being part of a formal teaching session. As an example, Kapsalis quotes a male physician who was told as a medical student, by his male supervisor, that 'during your first 70 pelvic exams, the only anatomy you'll feel is your own'. Over a decade later, a major review of the teaching of pelvic examinations concluded that the 'psychological impact' on the learner was not well explored in the literature. Little seems to have changed.

What does get discussed at great length in medical journals is the vexed issue of students practising on women who have been given a general anaesthetic prior to gynaecological surgery. Up until the early 1970s this was just how things were done, and questions weren't raised in the literature. In a paternalistic vein, arguments were made that women's modesty was protected by examining them when they were unconscious. Then, with the steady increase in the number of female medical students coupled with the growth of the feminist movement, this time-honoured way of teaching students began to be called into question. The central issue was that of consent; whilst the women would have consented to a surgical procedure, and might even have agreed to have a medical student present in theatre, they were never asked to give explicit consent for medical students to undertake an intimate examination of their body that had nothing whatsoever to do with their treatment.

Since the late 1970s, this issue has been debated at great length in medical journals and, from time to time, even makes national newspaper headlines. Attitudes of the general public have clearly moved on, with recent patient surveys indicating that the overwhelming majority of women expect to be asked before medical students are allowed to practise intimate examinations on them when they have had a general anaesthetic. But in many countries the old ways continue. For example, a survey published in 2011 of two medical schools in the UK and one in Australia found that, despite the existence in all three schools of explicit policies stressing the importance of gaining valid consent, students still found themselves in situations where they were being asked to conduct intimate examinations without consulting the patients.

The authors of the 2011 study highlighted the conflict between, on the one hand, patient expectations and societal norms, and on the other the 'weak ethical climate' in the clinical workplace, where examining anaesthetised women without their explicit consent continues. Although the authors don't unpick what's 'weak' about the workplace ethics in any detail, I would argue that one of the relevant factors is the systemic denial that intimate examinations have anything whatsoever to do with sex. An example of this would be the comment following the publication of an article in the *British Medical Journal* about the need to gain informed consent: 'This article is dangerous in that it isolates vaginal or rectal examinations as being intimate examinations.'

As a patient, I have different feelings when a doctor examines my vagina or rectum than I do when they look at my hands or feet. When it comes to sex, all body parts are equal, but some body parts are more equal than others.

Similarly, in 2009 there was online fury following the publication in a Canadian medical journal of an article entitled 'The other side of the speculum'. In the article, medical student Brent Thoma described his discomfort when performing a vaginal examination of a patient. Thoma was widely criticised for writing openly about his feelings, whilst other doctors criticised the journal for publishing the article in the first place. A lone voice was that of a female doctor who had this to say:

> Young men and women are still sexual beings as well as medical students, yet where in the curriculum do they have the opportunity to ask about the 'what ifs?' of medical examinations and procedures.

The answer for many students and junior doctors would seem to be 'nowhere'.

In a way, it's a bit like Hans Christian Andersen's story of the Emperor's New Clothes. The medical profession sets out to deny that intimate examinations have anything to do with sex. And just as it took a small boy standing on the side of the crowd to voice the obvious fact that the Emperor was naked, it took a psychiatrist – someone who stood outside the specialty of obstetrics and gynaecology – to write about students' fears of sexual arousal when examining women's vaginas. In an unusually candid academic article, an American psychiatrist, Julius Buchwald, described how the first pelvic examination was 'a kind of initiation rite, with clear sexual undercurrents'. Buchwald went on to say that students' fears of a sexual reaction to the patient tended not to be offered spontaneously.

Instead, the issue was raised after other anxieties had first been voiced, and usually in response to the seminar leader asking specifically about such fears.

Buchwald was writing in the late 1970s – but it would be wrong to think that things had changed much. Just as Buchwald highlighted how medical students used jokes when uncomfortable sexual feelings were discussed, a similar observation was made in a 2014 study in Australia. Very recently, a professor of obstetrics in London who teaches medical ethics told me that jokes are still used to mask feelings of sexual anxiety. As an example, she described a recent incident told to her in a seminar by a medical student. The (female) medical student was shadowing a male junior doctor in A & E, and she overheard him turn to his (male) colleague and say, 'That patient needs a tube.' In response, the student asked whether it was a bronchoscopy or endoscopy that the patient needed, and to her amazement this provoked uncontrolled laughter on the part of the two junior doctors. Eventually one turned to her and said, 'Not tube – T.U.B.E. – Totally Unnecessary Breast Examination.'

The student was left feeling humiliated that she had needed the acronym to be spelt out, and furious that her two more senior colleagues had been eyeing up talent in the A & E waiting area. Yet she hadn't voiced her upset until examples of professionally dubious practice were discussed in the context of the medical ethics seminar.

*

Freud, in his *Jokes and Their Relation to the Unconscious*, was the first to explore how jokes, alongside dreams and slips of the tongue, bear the traces of repressed desire. The whole tenor of medical training disallows explicit acknowledgement of sexual feelings on the part of the medical student or junior doctor. It's hardly surprising, then, that such feelings often get repackaged as jokes.

In the past year or so I have talked to doctors from all sorts of different specialties. My broad conclusion hasn't shifted: that medical education is in denial about doctors being sexual beings. Whilst a few colleagues have had training on how to cope with sexualised behaviour from patients, almost none had been part of a formal or informal discussion on what to do with their own sexual feelings. The exception to this rule was a GP colleague, who reminded me that a patient's attraction to a doctor is quite frequently discussed in a so-called 'Balint Group'. This GP went on to say that doctors rarely talked about their own attraction to patients in these groups, but sometimes alert group members reflected back to a colleague that it sounded as if patient–doctor sexual attraction wasn't only happening in one direction.

Balint Groups are not new – they were started in London by two psychoanalysts, Michael and Enid Balint, in the 1950s. In a typical Balint Group, six to twelve doctors, together with one or two leaders, meet on a regular basis. The leaders may come from different professional backgrounds (psychoanalysts, psychologists or doctors) and will have received training in group facilitation. The purpose of the group is to help doctors explore and better understand any uncomfortable feelings they have following a consultation with a particular patient.

Discussion within the group is entirely confidential and is not recorded, summarised or reported back to anybody outside the room. The meetings tend to last between one and a half and two hours, which gives participants an opportunity to discuss an individual consultation in great depth, and one case discussion may last for forty-five minutes. There is none of the feeling of rush that pervades much of clinical training. As one participant explained:

> You leave the group relieved and renewed about your dilemma because you learn to re-examine and redefine your role with this challenging patient through the eyes and ears and hearts of your colleagues. Inevitably the issues discussed relate to other members of the group, and they too leave with added insights.

The method has now spread to over twenty-two countries across the world and doctors throughout Europe, the Americas, Australia, New Zealand, and even Russia and China, take part in these groups. Although Balint Groups were originally set up to support GPs, they are now used by different medical specialties (psychiatry, palliative care) as well as in other healthcare professions such as nursing and psychology.

The Balints introduced the metaphor of the doctor as 'drug'; in other words, patients don't respond only to the medications that they are prescribed; they also respond to how the doctor treats them, as people. Instead of focusing on what is medically wrong with the patient, in a Balint

Group the relationship between the clinician and the patient takes centre stage. Clinicians are also asked to present a case in a particular way; they tell the 'story' of the patient consultation, focusing on their own feelings and the response of the patient. The clinician doesn't have the patient's notes in front of them, or printouts from the computer, instead they tell the story from memory. Group leaders encourage participants to bring those cases where the clinician has been left with uncomfortable feelings which linger long after the end of the consultation.

Both as a group member, and also as a co-leader, I have heard colleagues use the safety of the Balint Group to discuss potentially embarrassing sexual stuff. Once I was part of a temporary group formed over a three-day Balint training conference. The group that I was allocated to mostly consisted of Icelandic GP trainees. It was a fascinating three days; not only did these young Icelandic doctors have an exceptional use of English, but they also shed light on aspects of medical practice that I had never before heard voiced.

Many of these GP trainees were working in the small communities where they had grown up, and the cases they brought to the group highlighted the different problems that this could cause. As a young woman in your thirties, how can you best manage a consultation that starts with the patient reminding you that he remembers how cute you looked when you were still in nappies? How can you find a sexual partner in a small community when all the men you get introduced to are patients at the practice where you work? There's only one practice in town, so if you are attracted to a patient, is it ethical to ask them to see another GP in the practice, and then begin a sexual relationship?

Balint Groups provide an ideal place to raise the full range of feelings that can arise when one person cares for another. I wondered how Peter's career might have panned out if he had been part of a Balint Group. Maybe he would have used the group to discuss his discomfort with examining male bodies. And maybe he wouldn't have ended up in the highly acute specialty of obstetrics, and instead could have trained as a GP a decade earlier. Unfortunately, Balint Groups are thin on the ground, and only a tiny proportion of medical students or junior doctors get to benefit from the supportive, non-judgemental space they provide.

But if a doctor can't discuss sexual issues related to their work with their supervisors, and most don't have the opportunity to attend a Balint Group, where else can they turn?

I suppose a medical student or doctor could take a look at the advice given by their regulatory organisation to see if it casts any light on the matter. In the UK, medical practice is regulated by the General Medical Council (GMC), but guidelines published by this organisation wouldn't take you very far. This becomes clear when you compare what the GMC has to say about sexual boundaries with the Medical Council of New Zealand's advice on the same issue. Both sets of guidelines kick off in a similar vein. The GMC document published in 2013 states that:

Trust is the foundation of the doctor–patient partnership. Patients should be able to trust that their doctor will behave professionally towards them during consultations and not see them as a potential sexual partner.

Parallel guidance from New Zealand published a few years earlier is:

> The Council rejects the view that changing social standards require a less stringent approach. Only the highest standard is acceptable and the professional doctor–patient relationship must be one of absolute confidence and trust.

Not much difference there, with both professional bodies emphasising the centrality of trust. But the New Zealand guidelines also include a couple of simple, insightful statements:

> It is important to remember that doctors and patients have the same emotions and feelings as any other people. It is not uncommon for two people who meet in a professional setting to feel attracted to each other.
>
> Judgement on your behaviour is not based on the attraction you feel towards a patient but how you respond to this attraction.

At no point in the GMC document is the possibility raised that a doctor could feel attracted to a patient – and that they won't be judged for their feelings, but for their response in relation to the attraction. This omission becomes all the more surprising when you see how the GMC has failed to incorporate the findings of a national research project on sexual boundary violations in healthcare. And what makes it even more extraordinary is that the research project was commissioned by the Council for Healthcare Regulatory Excellence (CHRE), an umbrella organisation that oversees the work of the GMC as well as eight other healthcare regulatory bodies (nurses, pharmacists, etc.).

In 2008 the CHRE published a set of three documents: a clear statement on the responsibilities of healthcare professionals; an extensive literature review; and a series of recommendations on how best to train professionals in order to minimise boundary violations. This work was commissioned by the Department of Health in response to a series of inquiries into serious breaches of sexual boundaries by healthcare professionals. It was carried out in consultation with patient groups, professional bodies and health profession regulators including the General Medical Council. In the published documents, the possibility that a practitioner could be attracted to a patient is made explicit:

> If a healthcare professional is sexually attracted to a patient and is concerned that it may affect their professional relationship, they should ask for help and advice from a colleague or appropriate professional body, in order to decide on the most professional course of action to take.
>
> If a healthcare professional is asked for advice by a colleague who feels attracted to a patient or carer but has not acted inappropriately, they do not have a professional duty to inform anyone.

Students must be taught that there is nothing unusual or abnormal about having sexualised feelings towards certain patients, but that failing to identify these feelings and acting on them is likely to result in serious consequences for their patients and *themselves*.

All three reports were published before the GMC wrote its current statements about sexual boundaries. But the GMC's guidelines (unlike those of its Antipodean counterpart) contain no mention of the possibility that a doctor could ever feel attracted to a patient. In UK medicine at least, it seems as if doctors are not allowed to have sexual feelings towards those they treat, ever. Despite the fact that a national research project concluded that brushing these issues under the carpet *increases* the risk of sexual boundaries being breached, the topic is written out of the guidelines. So much for evidence-based medical education.

*

Shortly after setting up the Careers Unit, a doctor requested an urgent appointment. Whilst he told me in the session that he had failed to complete his GP training, he omitted to say that he was being investigated by the GMC, following the death of a patient, and that he had significant conditions attached to his licence to practise. After this experience, we routinely checked every doctor's listing on the open access GMC register, prior to their first appointment.

On a number of occasions I have seen doctors whose registration with the GMC was subject to the following conditions:

a. Except in life-threatening emergencies, you must not carry out consultations with female patients, without a chaperone present.

b. You must keep a log detailing every case where you have carried out a consultation with such a patient, which must be signed by the chaperone.

c. You must keep a log detailing every case where you have carried out a consultation with such a patient in a life-threatening emergency, without a chaperone present.

Typically doctors who have these sorts of conditions attached to their registration have been subject to a complaint from one or more female patients that they have been examined inappropriately. If the police are involved, and the doctor finds themselves charged with a sexual offence, even an acquittal in court won't necessarily protect them from having conditions placed on their registration. In court, the jury is instructed to apply the criminal standard of proof, that the prosecution has established the doctor's guilt 'beyond all reasonable doubt'. But in a Fitness to Practise tribunal, the panel has to apply the less stringent civil standard, namely, that 'on the balance of probabilities' the account of the patient was preferred over the account of the doctor. This crucial difference between 'beyond all reasonable doubt' and 'on the balance of probabilities' can sound the death knell to a doctor's medical career.

Often the proceedings drag on for an exceedingly long time. It's not unusual for it to take nearly a year from the point a doctor is charged, to the case being heard in a criminal court.

That's long enough. Then a subsequent Fitness to Practise tribunal during which conditions may get imposed on a doctor's registration, and any subsequent appeal can drag on for two years or more. Technically, if a doctor has conditions imposed (as opposed to suspension or erasure from the medical register) they can work as a doctor, as long as the conditions are met. In practice these doctors can find themselves in occupational limbo.

As a woman (and the mother of a daughter), I can imagine how horrible it would be if one thought that the doctor who was examining one's body was deriving sexual pleasure from the experience. It's stressful enough to let a stranger touch one's body in places that one otherwise reserves for a lover (or lets nobody touch). So I am not in any way condoning the behaviour of a doctor who attempts to obtain sexual gratification from their patients. I would also want to feel certain that the GMC had placed conditions of sufficient stringency on a doctor's practice so that future patients would never be left feeling violated, following a medical examination.

But I can also imagine some young doctors – particularly if they are sexually inexperienced – being tasked with carrying out an examination of a woman's body. Nobody is around – it's just the doctor and the patient in a cubicle. It felt different when these doctors had to examine a woman as a medical student. Back then there were a number of people watching over them, assessing what they were doing. Here it was just the doctor and the patient. Perhaps at this point there is an almost imperceptible change in the doctor' breathing or his hand seems to linger longer or stray further than the patient expects.

The patient has some sense that the doctor is not as detached as he should be and that something isn't quite right. Understandably, the patient feels that the trust she placed in the doctor has been abused. They would probably deem it necessary to lodge a formal complaint – and they would be right. Yet at the same time, I can't help but feel sadness about some of these young doctors.

On some level, they might well be aware that there is a problem. They note the frisson of excitement when they walk into a cubicle and find that the patient is a young woman – particularly if she is good-looking. And these doctors may be aware that the excitement increases when a clinical reason requires an internal examination. They know that they shouldn't be having these feelings. But they have no idea what to do about them.

At no stage in their training has anybody ever discussed the possibility that they might find aspects of examining a patient's body sexually exciting. The whole topic is taboo. They have read the GMC guidelines and know that doctors are not allowed to have relationships with patients, and that doctors mustn't use their privileged access to patients' bodies for their own sexual ends. But despite the explicit recommendation in the CHRE review that trainees should be taught that there is nothing unusual or abnormal about developing sexualised feelings towards patients and that it is acting on these feelings that is problematic – the GMC guidelines fail to mention that this could ever happen. Thus doctors in this position think that they alone have these feelings. They have no idea where to turn for help.

So they continue examining patients, keeping their shameful secrets to themselves until there is a complaint. And then the career they have dedicated themselves to for well over a decade comes crashing down. Any savings that they have get used up during the three-year period that it takes to complete the GMC proceedings. In theory the GMC conditions allow them to continue working but the harsh reality is that often it proves impossible to find a clinical setting where the conditions can be met.

When doctors with these sorts of conditions come to see me, I try to encourage them to explore options beyond medicine. But typically they counter this suggestion, pointing out that they have been acquitted of a crime and the GMC has kept them on the medical register, so why should they give up their dream of returning to medicine? But sometimes months have turned into years, and despite endless meetings, and sporadic hopes that a given hospital would offer them a job, each possible lead evaporates.

*

If the possibility of a doctor being aroused by a patient has never been discussed during one's training, how can young doctors seek out a trusted older colleague and talk about any sexual feelings that they may experience when carrying out intimate examinations? And as long as the taboo surrounding this issue remains in place, doctors will b denied opportunities to talk about their feelings and crucially – to put strategies in place so that their sexual desires aren't enacted when they are alone in the consulting room with a female patient.

There's also the impact of the regulatory process itself. Every medical system needs a way of holding doctors accountable, in order to protect the well-being of patients. This issue is not new. Four hundred years before the birth of Christ, Hippocrates recognised that doctors had privileged access to patients' bodies, leading to the danger that this can be exploited for sexual ends. But when we look at our 21st-century solution to the problem, it's hard to conclude that we have got it quite right.

Following a spate of suicides of doctors who were subject to GMC investigations, an internal review was commissioned which published its findings in late 2014. Amongst the report's many recommendations were the need to reduce the length of time it takes to complete an investigation and the importance of assisting – in a compassionate way – doctors who are being investigated. The following year the GMC commissioned a specialist service to provide confidential emotional support to any doctor involved in a Fitness to Practise case. These developments would have helped some of the doctors I've encountered.

Maybe the arcane details of specialty training regulations in the UK are particularly hard to navigate. But I suspect that doctors in other countries face comparable challenges once they have been reported to the regulator. Across the English-speaking world, only the GMC has published data on the psychological impact of being the subject of a Fitness to Practise investigation. As a national body, the GMC is in a stronger position to undertake this sort of research than the regulatory organisations in the USA and Canada, where disciplining doctors takes place at the state rather than the national level. Little is known about what happens to doctors in these countries who end up falling foul of the regulator. But I don't imagine that their stories have happy endings.

5

Role Reversal

S arah had planned to conceive her first child in December so that it would be born the following September. She had read that children with birthdays at the beginning of the school year tended to do better academically and she wanted to ensure that she gave her child the best start in life. But four years later, with no baby in sight despite a range of different fertility treatments, Sarah didn't care what month she conceived; she just wanted a baby.

In our sessions together it became clear that her inability to conceive was overshadowing everything else. She described herself as somebody who liked order and control in her life and planned everything meticulously. Whether it was revising for postgraduate exams or preparing for her wedding, Sarah needed to know that she had left nothing to chance. Sadly, she .ad to learn that even with the best fertility treatment on offer, r baby project could still fail. And she didn't have the option 'mmersing herself in her work as a distraction from the pain of infertility. Babies *were* her work, as Sarah was an obstetrician.

Every hour of her working day Sarah was surrounded by women who were either expecting babies or were in the process of giving birth to them. The only exception was the infertility clinic where she had to talk to patients about the different treatment options, all of which had failed to work for her. When her infertility patients became pregnant she longed to be the patient rather than doctor. When they failed to get pregnant it not only reminded her of her own childlessness, but also made her feel useless. A doctor who couldn't protect her patients from the pain she was feeling herself.

When Sarah first came to see me she felt trapped. She was in her sixth year of specialty training as an obstetrician, had long since passed all her postgraduate exams, and in a couple of years' time would be eligible to apply for a permanent post as a consultant. Yet the prospect of delivering other women's babies for the rest of her life, if she herself couldn't have one, filled her with dread.

One might have imagined that as Sarah's colleagues were all obstetricians who had treated infertile patients they would have been kind and sympathetic to her predicament. But they weren't. The prevailing response from her supervisor seemed to be that she should 'pull herself together, and concentrate on her patients'. What made this even more galling was that she knew from colleagues that this particular consultant had needed IVF treatment to become pregnant.

A similar thing happened in Sarah's annual review meeting. The whole procedure left her feeling bitterly disappointed.

the training system; nobody on the panel accepted that her struggle to conceive should have had any impact on how she was feeling about her career. Instead they implied that she was lazy, or unmotivated, or making a fuss about a minor matter. She later found out that two senior consultants on the panel had also been through IVF, yet neither had come to her defence.

I couldn't give Sarah what she most wanted in life. But by the end of our sessions, two things became clearer for her. First, she came to understand that the pain she experienced at work wasn't a sign of weakness. It would be extremely cruel to walk somebody who was starving through a supermarket stocked full of food without letting them eat. In the same way, to expect a young woman who was trying to come to terms with her own infertility to be surrounded by pregnant women and babies and just be able to 'pull herself together and get on with her work' was both heartless and unrealistic.

The second thing we were able to do in the sessions was to come up with a Plan B – an escape route – should Sarah feel at some time in the future that she needed to change career. The small number of consultants who were able to give credence to her distress had suggested that the obvious thing was for her to retrain as a GP. But Sarah instinctively felt that the GP route was the wrong option, and I agreed.

Prior to her difficulty getting pregnant, Sarah had loved the drama of the delivery suite, where you are always working alongside lots of other colleagues. Being on her own in a GP surgery held no appeal. She had also enjoyed the fact that pregnancy was a time-limited condition with a definite end. In contrast, with specialties that she had encountered earlier in her career, she had found it depressing to treat lots of patients with chronic illnesses, often with poor prognoses. If she trained as a GP, her surgery would be full of patients with long-term conditions which had no quick cure.

Through our discussions Sarah decided that, should she need to switch in future, emergency medicine would be a better Plan B. This option would give her lots of colleagues and lots of drama, and – perhaps most important of all – with a four-hour limit on being treated: patients in A and E either become the responsibility of clinical colleagues in other hospital departments, or they are discharged back to the care of their GP, who is responsible for providing life-long care.

That doctors, or their family members, should be inflicted with the same conditions as their patients isn't surprising. But what *was* surprising in Sarah's case was the way her supervisors made her feel that she was at fault for experiencing distress. Somehow, as a doctor, she was expected to be able to rise above any upset. Other doctors respond to this expectation by feeling that there is something wrong with them if they can't push their feelings to one side and just get on with their work. This was what happened to a paediatrician called Orla who came to see me shortly before she was due to start a neonatal placement.

Orla had recently experienced, for the third time, a late pregnancy loss, and she was dreading the prospect of caring for newborn infants. She hadn't countenanced the possibility that her rotation could be altered, or that she could request some time out of training to recover from her recurrent miscarriages. Luckily the clinician in charge of paediat training was extremely sympathetic, and Orla's neonatal rotation was changed. But when I first suggested it to her, Orla felt that such a switch would only be granted in much more severe situations; she had no sense that most women would find caring for neonates challenging if they had recently lost three pregnancies.

*

At least Orla knew why the prospect of working with neonates felt unbearable. I've also encountered doctors who have repressed any conscious connection between events in their personal lives and their feelings about work – which was what happened to Jack.

In our first session, Jack told me he wanted to leave medicine. We talked through his career history; when he had first thought about medicine, his experience at medical school and how things had panned out once he started working as a doctor. Nothing he told me cast any light on his current dissatisfaction at work. Puzzled, I asked him about his current placement. Were his supervisors supportive? How were his colleagues? This line of enquiry also led nowhere, as he liked all of his current team.

'Tell me a bit about your family,' I said. 'Is there anything going on at home that might be having an impact on your work?'

Jack let out an audible sigh, paused, and looked down at the floor.

'My mum was diagnosed with breast cancer three months ago. She's responding well to the treatment, but it's hard to find time to visit her as much as I would like.'

Jack was rotating through different medical specialties, and currently was working with cancer patients. Extraordinary as it sounds, he hadn't made the conscious link between his mother's illness and his growing unhappiness at work. Once we started to talk about it, he realised that when patients responded poorly to treatment, he felt extremely anxious. Perhaps that was how his mother's cancer would progress in future. And irrespective of their prognoses, he resented spending time with other people's mothers rather than his own. When Jack gave voice to his fears about his mother's illness and seeing how being surrounded by patients with cancer constantly reminded him of her, his urge to flee medicine felt much less acute.

*

The challenge that doctors face when they themselves become ill isn't just that their patients remind them of their own health concerns, which makes it hard for them to take refuge in their work. Far bigger than this issue of reminders is that of incompatible roles. Like the binary alternatives zero and one, the culture within medicine often positions patient and doctor as mutually exclusive categories. You can be one, or the other – but never both together.

Psychiatrist Robert Klitzman had a sister who died in the attack on the World Trade Center on September 11, 2001. A few months later he became seriously depressed – although he resisted the diagnosis initially. Through this personal experience he became interested in how doctors respond when they face a significant illness, and once he had recovered and returned to clinical practice he set about researching this topic. Th extreme difficulty of being both a doctor *and* a patient is one of the major themes that emerged.

For example, Jessica, a paediatrician in his study, who was being treated for cancer, described how her oncologist talked to her as if she were a colleague rather than a patient:

> Because I was a doctor, he would talk to me about his other patients. 'I have a patient just like you. She looks like you: same age, and has the same exact tumour. She's in the hospital.' So of course I say, 'How's she doing?' He says, 'She's dying.'

Of course it's not inappropriate for colleagues to discuss the similarity between two cases – this happens all the time. But even though Jessica was a colleague, it was insensitive in the extreme to draw her attention to this other patient. One can't imagine that the doctor would have made this comparison to a patient who wasn't also a colleague. Jessica, and many of the other doctors in Klitzman's study, encountered less than optimal care because their treating physicians approached them as if they were colleagues rather than patients.

But Klitzman's analysis makes it clear that the root cause is more complex than that of insensitive physicians. Many of the doctors in Klitzman's study described how difficult they found it to relinquish the role of doctor and assume that of a patient. So, for example, Dan, an oncologist with metastatic lung cancer, described how:

> The hospital staff have seen me over the years and know who I am. It's very strange to sit there in a hospital gown . . . When

I go for my scans, I bring along a pair of [theatre] scrubs, and change into scrubs, rather than into one of their sets of patient pyjamas which, because of my girth, don't fit me.

Dan may have rationalised this decision as relating to his size. But by choosing clothes that doctors wear at work (theatre scrubs) rather than more neutral attire (a tracksuit, for example), he was simultaneously reminding people of his professional status. Non-medical patients don't have access to theatre scrubs.

So doctors, when ill, often struggle to be seen as patients, in the same way that doctors treating other doctors might respond to them as colleagues rather than sick patients. Both parties contribute to the difficulty of inhabiting a space where somebody could be *both* a doctor and a patient at the same time.

Sarah, the obstetrician who couldn't conceive, was viewed by her colleagues as a doctor rather than a patient. I cannot imagine that other patients these colleagues were treating in their infertility clinics would have been told that they should just pull themselves together and stop worrying about whether or not they would conceive. But Sarah was a doctor and therefore, in their eyes, shouldn't be vulnerable to the distress experienced by non-medical patients.

In contrast, Orla's supervisors understood that working with newborn babies so soon after losing three pregnancies could pose an intolerable emotional burden. In this case, it was Orla who struggled to allow herself to assume the role of patient. She was gentle and kind, and I am sure that she was a highly empathic paediatrician. When supporting parents after one of her paediatric patients died, I imagine she was well aware of the pain that these parents suffered. But when faced with her own losses, it was hard for her to ask for help.

*

Sadly Sarah and Orla are far from unique. I have seen many doctors whose careers have been derailed by health issues. Sometimes their problems were compounded by their own difficulties in accepting that they were unwell. At other times, enormous distress has been caused by the intransigence of their supervising consultants – all of whom were doctors – in making any allowances for the fact that they were ill.

One doctor, Amy, whom I only saw a couple of times, had left medicine a few years earlier, and was attempting to return to clinical training. Amy had been diagnosed with insulin-dependent diabetes shortly before her medical school finals. Although she passed all her examinations, once she started working as a junior hospital doctor, the stress of the job, combined with working nights and irregular mealtimes, meant that she couldn't keep her diabetes well controlled. As a doctor Amy knew only too well the longer-term implications of poor diabetic control (blindness, heart disease, kidney failure, amongst other conditions), and she became terrified that by continuing to work she was jeopardising her future well-being. So she left her job as a doctor.

For a few years Amy worked in a research lab without any responsibility for patients. During this period she got used to managing her illness, and eventually was able to achieve reasonable diabetic control. She then successfully applied for a post that allowed her to complete her foundation training, and at the point when she came to see me she was about to apply for a place on a GP training scheme.

What prompted Amy's request for a meeting was that one of her supervisors had advised her to lie on her application form. Instead of giving the true reason for her time away from clinical practice – that she had been struggling to get her diabetes under control – the supervisor suggested she should come up with some other story. Perhaps she could say that family members had been ill. Amy was particularly upset by her supervisor's comment that, if she talked about her diabetes, she would never get a place on a GP training scheme.

My view was that Amy had been given lousy advice. Leaving aside the fact that there is legislation in place to protect an applicant from discrimination on the grounds of health, there were two major flaws in her supervisor's suggestion. First, if, for whatever reason, the lie had been discovered, Amy's application would have been thrown out. She might even have been reported to the GMC. Honesty is a core professional value in medicine – and indeed in all other professions. Advising somebody to lie is encouraging them to commit professional suicide.

Second, chronic illnesses including diabetes are increasingly managed by GPs, rather than by hospital doctors. Patients with chronic illnesses also have to manage complex treatment regimens at home, and problems with non-adherence are rife. It's not always easy to take medications according to a strict timetable, or stick to diet and exercise recommendations. Amy had personal experience of making changes in her life in order to accommodate the demands of a lifelong illness. Rather than hiding her diagnosis on her application form, she could turn it round to her advantage and talk about what she had learnt, and how she would use her experience to support patients when they struggled with different chronic conditions. Amy didn't lie on her application form or at interview. And she was successfully appointed to a GP training scheme.

*

Being accepted as a doctor with diabetes is one thing, but many of the doctors in Klitzman's study talked about the stigma attached to psychiatric symptoms. For example, Jessica, the paediatrician with cancer, became depressed during her treatment. When this happened, she felt blamed by her colleagues: 'Cancer's not your fault. You can't help it. But doctors view mental illness as your own fault. I felt it in conversations about other people: a lessening of respect for the person who had it.'

Another doctor in Klitzman's study, Ernie, had been diagnosed with Huntington's Disease – an incurable genetic condition with increasingly severe neurological and psychiatric symptoms. He had this to say: 'I have not faced any discrimination from Huntington's Disease. But the hospital was not nice about the depression: they actually were going to fire me!'

Not surprisingly, given these sorts of responses, doctors in Klitzman's study who experienced psychiatric symptoms talked about the difficulty of admitting (to themselves, and to others) that they had become mentally unwell.

Over the years I have spoken to doctors diagnosed with a number of illnesses, including cancer, MS, epilepsy, narcolepsy, rheumatoid arthritis, diabetes, Crohn's Disease, lupus, schizo-phrenia, bipolar disorder, and depression. Whilst many have struggled to progress their medical careers, given the difficulty of being both a doctor and a patient, doctors diagnosed with psychiatric conditions have undoubtedly had the hardest time of all.

As one psychiatrist told me, following his admission to a psychiatric ward:

> The other patients were always moaning about the psychiatrists who treated them. I didn't want any of them to know what my job was. But the psychiatrists treating me saw me as a patient rather than a colleague – I didn't belong with them either.

After a pause, he continued: 'On the ward I couldn't be either a patient or a psychiatrist. And there was no way that I could be both.'

*

How can we best understand the impossibility of being allowed to be both a doctor *and* a patient at the same time?

The most compelling answer is that the doctor–patient split serves an important psychological function. On a daily basis, doctors encounter distress, disease and death. Doctors are mortal, as are the people they love. So any of the difficult things they see in their patients could happen in future to them, their families or their friends. (Indeed, as we have seen in previous chapters, some of these tragedies may already have happened in their lives, which might be one of the reasons why they were drawn to medicine in the first place.) Positioning themselves as 'other' than their patients happens unconsciously, and assists doctors in going about their work without being psychologically overwhelmed by anxiety.

The notion that people can respond to extreme anxiety by resorting unconsciously to these sorts of defensive strategies might sound far-fetched. But how else can we explain the fact that the doctors who had themselves experienced fertility difficulties were the least sympathetic to Sarah's plight? The simple explanation is that Sarah's infertility reminded them that they too had once been treated for the same condition. This reminder was far from welcome as it made them feel vulnerable – so they reacted with particular hostility as they tried to distance themselves from Sarah's experience.

It's also important to acknowledge that the fantasy of being categorically different from one's patients is often institutionally reinforced from the very beginning of medical training. The author Michael Crichton isn't the only doctor who has commented on the place that human dissection plays in this respect: 'An important part of the dissection laboratory is that it requires students to break taboos surrounding the desecration of human remains . . . such an act has the effect of setting the medical student apart from others,' concluded two researchers.

Writing about his experience as a medical student, psychiatrist and psychoanalyst Norman Straker had this to say:

> I remember my first day of medical school as a young medical
> student with horror. We were casually introduced to our cadavers

without any preparation or discussion. My first cut into the cadaver was the first of many traumatic experiences in medical school that changed me. I was being prepared psychologically to be an objective doctor . . . I now believe that this frightening experience with no preparation began the unconscious psychological defensive split between the patient and me. Cadavers, our first patients, were made very distinct from us, the healthy 'immortal medical students.' Our defense against death, 'our specialness,' was being established.

Norman Straker was describing what happened forty years ago. I doubt whether this institutional neglect of the potential emotional impact of dissection would happen nowadays. As an example, Sabine Hildebrant, a researcher based at Harvard Medical School, has outlined a range of different strategies that need to be incorporated into the anatomy curriculum, in order to prepare students for dissection. Her suggestions include identifying those students who might find the experience particularly stressful, pre-course meetings, team reflection in the lab with faculty feedback, and a memorial service organised by students for faculty, students and donor families. Other medical schools – particularly some of the newer ones – have entirely abandoned the use of human dissection as a way of teaching anatomy. Times have moved on.

But despite all these changes, in those schools that use dissection, the cadaver is still routinely referred to as the 'first patient'. And whilst on the one hand it could be argued that this reminds students of the need to treat the cadaver with respect, on the other hand, as Norman Straker suggests, it also reinforces the idea that doctors and patients are categorically different.

*

I was once invited to sit in on an interview preparation workshop that a consultant organised for foundation trainees in his hospital. It was a 'twilight' session – held at the end of the working day after doctors on the day shift had handed over to their night-shift colleagues. I remember the doctors coming into the teaching room in the hospital education centre in successive waves – they couldn't leave the different wards around the hospital until somebody had come to relieve them. And I also remember being touched by their delight at finding that tea and biscuits had been provided at the back of the room. Tiny examples of being cared for or nourished by the training system are often in short supply for junior doctors.

Although these foundation doctors would have had times in the week when they were brought together for training, most of the week they would have been separated, spread thinly across the different hospital wards. They were eager to catch up with each other's news, and before the session started there were noisy and animated conversations going on within the group. And a lot of laughter.

The furniture in the room made it clear that there was going to be a mock-interview. At the front was a table with two chairs facing each other – one for the interviewer, and one for the interviewee. Behind the interview table were rows of seats, arranged in such a way that the doctors could sit and observe.

'Let's get started,' said the consultant. 'Who is brave enough to go first?'

'I will,' answered one of the trainees.

I'd noticed this woman as she came in, cracking jokes with her colleagues. But it wasn't only her animated manner that had caught my eye – she was over a foot shorter than most of her colleagues. She suffered from dwarfism.

With some difficulty this trainee manoeuvred herself into the hot seat and the consultant kicked off with his first question.

'What makes you stand out as a doctor?' he asked.

The colour drained from the trainee's cheeks, and for a brief moment I thought she was going to cry. All eyes in the room were on this young woman and collectively we witnessed how the animation present a few minutes earlier, when she was laughing with her colleagues, seeped out of her body. As if temporarily frozen, she was unable to speak. A couple of seconds later, with obvious difficulty she regained her composure and started to answer the question.

It was painful to see this lively young woman rendered temporarily speechless in front of her colleagues. And why had the consultant been so clumsy with his choice of words? At the time I thought the consultant must have been unusually insensitive – somebody who spoke without first thinking about possible associations of the words he chose to use. But over the next few years when doctors with different physical and sensory disabilities came to see me, I learnt that such insensitivity was not uncommon.

Just like the consultant's in the mock-interview course, the comments were often thoughtless rather than deliberately cruel

So, for example, I've never forgotten one hearing-impaired doctor, Ian, who repeatedly had to ask his consultant on a ward round not to hold the patient's notes in a way that obscured her mouth. Day after day the consultant made it impossible for Ian to lip-read what she was saying. After yet another interminable ward round when he was left unclear what clinical tasks he needed to get on with, Ian reminded his consultant about his reliance on lip-reading.

'The trouble is, Ian, you're such an able doctor. We all forget that you lip-read,' said the consultant. 'Why don't you wear a badge saying "I'm Deaf"?'

Ian remained silent. Yet this insensitive comment, along-side the lack of provision of basic equipment such as a device to enable him to use the telephone on the ward, eroded his motivation to the point that he was considering leaving medi-cine. Luckily his next placement was completely different, and Ian was able to rediscover his enjoyment of clinical practice.

Other doctors with a range of physical and sensory impair-ments also told me about hospitals' failure to provide vital equipment. And this equipment that didn't materialise despite being requested wasn't multimillion-dollar kit – it was specialist chairs, or information printed in larger type. The sorts of accommodation that medical schools and hospital trusts were legally obliged to provide in order to be compliant with equality legislation. Doctors like Ian knew that they could have sought legal redress, but frequently they didn't want to be seen as difficult or demanding, so they just put up with inadequate (and legal) levels of support.

Sadly, alongside thoughtless comments and lack of necessary equipment, there were also examples of downright hostility. 'I don't know why you were ever allowed to come and work here,' was the greeting that one doctor with a physical disability received on her first day of a new job. Another was told within days of starting that 'this is never going to work out'. Faced with this type of response from her consultant, the trainee found herself unable to carry out straightforward procedures such as taking blood, which she had performed without any difficulty in her previous, far more supportive placement.

Little wonder then that some doctors tried to hide their disabilities, fearful of the impact these might have on their careers. I remember, in particular, a doctor with a progressive congenital visual impairment who hadn't told anybody at work about his slowly deteriorating eyesight. I managed to persuade him that even if he lost his sight entirely, there would still be jobs for him in health policy or health promotion, or in the pharmaceutical industry. But if it was discovered that he had been seeing patients without having an occupational health assessment of his vision, he risked a referral to the GMC, and possibly being struck off for a lack of professionalism. With that black mark against his name, establishing his career in a non-patient-facing role might prove far harder. Luckily he listened to me, and he agreed to go and see occupational health. His eyesight was judged to be good enough for clinical work, although provision was made to check it regularly in future. However, I've never forgotten the message he left on my answerphone, as he sat in the occupation health waiting room:

'Caroline, I'm frightened.'

*

Julie Madorsky, a physical medicine and rehabilitation specialist in California, was once teaching a group of medical students about the work opportunities for people with physical disabilities. A gowned patient was wheeled in, and it was explained that the patient had cerebral palsy (a neurological condition caused by problems in the parts of the brain responsible for controlling muscles) together with a speech impediment and severe ataxia (loss of full control of bodily movements). After Madorsky had taken the patient's history and carried out a physical examination, the patient was wheeled out and the medical students were asked to appraise his capacity for learning or employment. The collective opinion of the students was that the patient was severely disabled and could do a menial part-time job perhaps, but nothing more. The patient got dressed, returned to the classroom and was re-introduced as Dr Thomas Strax, Assistant Medical Director at a rehabilitation hospital in Pennsylvania. That was his position in real life.

If you had asked the medical students before the session about their views on employing patients with disabilities, I suspect that most of them would have talked about the importance of equality of opportunity. But faced with a patient with a significant physical impairment, they jumped to stereotypical assumptions about his intellectual and occupational potential.

I doubt that the medical students in that classroom ever forgot that session. I also imagine that Julie Madorsky was driven to carry out what some people might think of as an act of deception because of the intransigence of attitudes towards the disabled within the medical profession. She wrote: 'a constant refrain is that physicians, however educated and beneficent, are a steadfast impediment to bringing the disabled into medicine'.

Just like the doctor with dwarfism on the interview course, reports on the experience of doctors with physical and sensory disabilities are replete with examples of casual insensitivity. For example studies have detailed thoughtlessness in relation to anticipating problems with access – such as when a senior academic physician who was due to be honoured at an award ceremony found herself stranded in her wheelchair, at the bottom of a flight of steps into the hall. Then, as if her dignity hadn't already been compromised enough by having to be carried up the steps, she couldn't risk having any refreshments during the award ceremony because there was no wheelchair-accessible toilet.

A doctor in an American study who walked with crutches described how on the morning of his interview for an academic position at a prestigious medical school, the search committee chairman parked at the back of the garage, rather than dropping him off at the front door. 'I knew by 9.00,' reported the candidate. 'They were marching me back and forth from one building to another, just to prove to me it was the wrong place for me.'

Similarly, another doctor who relied on crutches described her first hospital post as 'an environment of isolation'. This doctor stressed that the lack of acceptance was not by patients or nursing staff, but by physicians.

So what's going on?

Just as doctors unconsciously position themselves in a separate category from the patients they treat, in order not to be overwhelmed by anxieties that they too could become sick, there is a tendency for able-bodied people to position themselves as 'other' than the disabled in order to avoid confronting the possibility that they, too, might one day join their ranks. To quote a writer on disability, Jenny Morris:

> It is fear and denial of the frailty, vulnerability, mortality and arbitrariness of human experience that deters us from confronting such realities. Fear and denial prompt the isolation of those who are disabled, ill or old as 'other', as 'not like us'.

But what does this mean for doctors with disabilities?

It means that they face a double whammy. Doctors are supposed to be uber-able, not disabled.

*

Unsurprisingly, doctors are reluctant to admit to having a disability. For example, a report by the BMA Equal Opportunities Committee in 2007 found that 'due to the culture within the medical profession, and the stigma attached to the term "disabled", there is a great deal of under-reporting of impairment by doctors'. More recently a study in a Scottish medical school reached a similar conclusion.

Some medical schools have introduced a 'card' scheme in order to empower students with disabilities or health conditions request appropriate support. The cards are authorised by the Dean of the Medical School and the specific wording is agreed between the student and relevant senior faculty. The idea is that the student hands the card to whoever is teaching them, who then ensures that necessary adjustments (such as allowing a student to sit down on a ward round) are made. This is all well and good but it says something about the unspeakable nature of illness and disability within medical training that such a scheme is necessary. Students can't simply go to faculty, have a frank and open discussion about their problems and expect that their needs will be taken into account. Instead they need a card authorised by the dean, before they will be listened to. And even then, some students were reluctant to use the card, and others encountered unresponsive teaching staff. Attitudes to illness and disability within the profession are hard to shift.

On paper, there are, of course, legal protections. In the UK, disabled doctors are protected by the 2010 Equality Act, which supersedes the earlier Disability Discrimination Act. In the US, the relevant legislation is the Americans with Disabilities Act of 1990. But like Ian (the hearing-impaired doctor whose consultant suggested he should wear a badge saying 'I'm Deaf'), most are reluctant to seek legal redress. Even when, in strict contravention of the law, necessary reasonable adjustments (such as the provision of special chairs, or hearing equipment) haven't been made – disabled doctors don't want to rock the boat.

Major institutional stakeholders such as the BMA and the GMC are, of course, aware of the legal requirements. In fac in the UK it was the introduction of the 2010 Equality Act t' prompted the GMC to commission a major review of health and disability in medical education and training. One of the issues considered by the review was the feasibility of granting disabled medical students exemptions from certain competencies, which would mean that they would graduate from medical school with restricted registration. The logic here is that currently medical students need to demonstrate basic competence in tasks such as skin suturing that they would never be called on to use in a number of different medical specialties (public health or psychiatry, for example). If somebody, by dint of a disability, couldn't suture skin, but wanted to go into psychiatry, why couldn't they be exempted from this and other such competencies at medical school, and be granted a form of registration which restricted their later career choices to specialties where suturing would never be needed?

The GMC review recognised that granting restricted registration might allow more disabled people to join the medical profession. But the review still concluded that this was not the best way forward. It gave a number of reasons: to begin with, in pressurised clinical environments somebody might be needed to carry out a duty that they had been exempted from; second, restricted registration might lead to stigmatisation of disabled doctors; and third, disabled students and trainees consulted in their focus groups were not in favour of granting exemptions.

Given the cultural antipathy within the profession towards disability, I would tend to agree that introducing restricted registration might – at least initially – increase the stigmatiation of doctors with disabilities. I can also see that it ight take some care and planning, if such a scheme were introduced, in order to ensure that at nights or at weekends, when staffing levels were reduced, a patient didn't need an urgent clinical task to be carried out that fell beyond the scope of the given doctor on duty. But paradoxically there is already good evidence that adjustments can be made without compromising the safety of patients. And where does this evidence come from?

The GMC.

The latest edition of a GMC publication entitled *Achieving Good Medical Practice: A Guide for Medical Students* states that:

> Students with blood-borne viruses can study medicine, but they may have restrictions on their clinical placements, must complete the recommended health screening before undertaking exposure-prone procedures, and will need to limit their medical practice when they graduate.

So on the one hand, the GMC rules that students with blood-borne viruses, such as hepatitis B and C, may, on graduation, need to avoid exposure-prone procedures and ask a colleague to take over, in order to ensure that they don't inadvertently infect a patient. On the other hand the GMC argues that offering disabled doctors restricted registration could cause problems in a busy clinical environment, if some doctors can't carry out certain procedures.

The GMC position simply doesn't stack up.

What about the GMC's argument that the disabled doctors in their focus groups didn't want restricted registration to be introduced?

That may be true for some doctors. But others like Jemma Saville would disagree.

*

Jemma Saville was diagnosed with dominant optic atrophy (loss of function of the optic nerve) during the second year of her medical degree. In a *BMJ* article in April 2008, Jemma was upbeat about her future career in medicine:

'My medical school has been very supportive,' she said. 'The staff have arranged extra teaching for me on subjects like anatomy, and provided presentations in large print so that I can read them with a magnifier. I want other students to know that, with adjustments, an impairment or disability does not necessarily rule out a career in medicine.'

Later on that year Jemma successfully sat her medical school finals, and graduated as a doctor. But she was then informed that there were no foundation jobs that could accommodate her visual impairment.

The following year, while she was still campaigning to be allowed to continue in medicine, Jemma's story was included in a BMA publication entitled *A Celebration of Disabled Doctors*. She remained optimistic:

I would still recommend medicine as a career! I do believe that it will take time, but I will get to practise as a doctor eventually, and when this happens, it will set a precedent for other graduates. Even with all the fighting, I loved my medical degree. Medicine is a wonderful mix of cience, practical work and, best of all, people. But I almost gave it up, because it's just such a struggle as a disabled person.

Jemma's next strategy was to petition the NHS to give her a foundation job (without which she couldn't progress to her eventual chosen specialty – psychiatry). On the petition website she had this to say:

> I don't want to perform clinical procedures which I am not competent to do, and I certainly would never put any patients at risk. I know what I can and can't do, and this is key to any doctor being safe. I believe that even with a visual impairment, I can be a very successful, inspirational doctor. I just need to be given the opportunity to prove this.

Jemma was never given that opportunity. In the end she gave up, and retrained as a teacher. When I contacted her, she had this to say:

'I'm actually very happy. I now have a hugely rewarding job which I love – teaching is my passion,' she told me. 'It's just a shame medicine couldn't offer me that.'

If Jemma had lived in the US, her story might have had a different ending.

Tim Cordes was born blind. In 1998, he applied to the University of Wisconsin Medical School. According to a clinician on the admission review committee, his application was exceptional, with extraordinarily high Medical College Admission Test scores, a near perfect undergraduate grade point average, and outstanding prior research experience antibiotics. Panel members assumed that every medical degree programme in the country would be fighting to get him – but they were wrong. Cordes applied to eight medical schools, but was turned down by the other seven. Only the University of Wisconsin was willing to offer him a place, and even there, some panel members were bitterly opposed to the idea of accepting a blind student. Sadly, opposition wasn't restricted to faculty members; on his first week, a fellow student sidled up to him in the canteen and asked, 'What are *you* doing here?'

In an article in the *Braille Monitor* in 2010, Cordes describes how he managed to complete his medical degree:

> I did anatomy by touch, feeling the nerves and muscles, doing some of the dissections. I was the guy who reached into the chest cavity up to my elbow to pull out our cadaver's lungs. When it came time for testing, I had the same test as everyone else, and felt and identified the muscles and nerves that way ... Much is made of the visual nature of medicine, and although we would love 100 per cent accessibility, the vast majority of information is easily accessible with speech software, electronic documents, CDs and the Internet. They don't tell you that, but it's true.

In addition to technical innovations, Tim was also helped by 'visual describers' – assistants who went through the clinical rotations of medical school with him, describing what they saw, and guiding him into the operating theatre while he held his sterile hands aloft to avoid contamination.

Cordes didn't only qualify as a doctor – he was also accepted on to an extremely competitive combined MD/PhD programme which trains practising clinicians to be scientific researchers. While working on his PhD analysing the structure of a bacterial protein, he devised a computer program to convert visual images of protein structure into sounds – going up and down the scale, and getting louder and softer, to explain the branching arms of the protein. This software is now available to help other visually impaired scientists.

But even with all these extraordinary achievements, Cordes still encountered resistance when applying for psychiatry residency programmes:

'I was interviewing at a residency in the north-east, and the chair of the department wanted to meet with me. After some pleasantries he said, "You know, I just don't get it. How are you going to know what's going on with a patient?"

'I paused, and then I said, "Well I know you're reading your email right now as you are talking to me." That opened a door.'

Eventually Cordes obtained a place on a residency, finished his training and is currently a psychiatrist in a Veterans Health Administration hospital, specialising in addictions. Dr Dean Krahn, the Head of Psychiatry at the hospital, has commented on the particular skill that Cordes brings to this work: 'Given that he can't see, I think that he's more attentive to everything you say . . . He listens closely for the sound of your breathing, the tone of your voice . . . He senses a lot about the patient and has a unique way of picking up on things other doctors might miss.'

Krahn then went on to describe why Cordes is especially attuned to treating veterans with addiction problems:

'There's a lot of pressure on people with addictions ... They're often told that they just need to change, that they need to overcome that hurdle in their lives. And their response? They'll say, "Doc, you don't know what it's like. It's not a hurdle I can just overcome. It's just too hard" ... But you know what? They tend to say that a lot less to Tim ... It's like his patients are thinking to themselves: "This guy's been blind since he was a little kid, and now he's a doctor. If he can do that, then I can stay sober today."'

*

Clearly Tim Cordes is an exceptional human being. At the same time, when we think about people with disabilities, we need to guard against a rhetoric of 'Anything is possible' or 'There is no such thing as "can't"'. Just as not everybody has the academic ability to train as a doctor, not all blind people could match Tim Cordes's achievements. Instead, we need to recognise the complexity and diversity of human life and avoid polarised thinking. To quote clinical psychologist Brian Watermeyer: 'Disabled people remain unknown within a view which constructs them – in an unreal manner – as heroic or helpless.'

If I think about Ian, or Jemma Saville, or any of the other doctors with disabilities whom I have encountered, I feel saddened that the culture of medicine has frequently failed to acknowledge their individual potential – or appreciate what they might be able to offer the profession. If Jemma Saville had lived the US, perhaps, like Tim Cordes, she would have been able to make use of her medical degree, and qualify as a psychiatrist. And if Tim Cordes had lived in the UK – he would never have been able to train as a doctor. What a loss. What a waste.

There is one point, however, with which I am in full agreement with the GMC, and that is the assertion that, if students with disabilities were offered restricted registration, 'the understanding of what it means to be "a doctor" could be completely changed'. Inadvertently, this statement gets to the heart of the matter. Restricted registration would allow doctors like Tim Cordes to qualify in the UK – a doctor who has no sight whatsoever. It would allow Thomas Strax – the wheelchair-bound physician with limited muscle control – to practise in the UK. It would allow people who have no hearing and communicate through a sign-language interpreter (as is happening in Canada) to join the profession. And countless others besides. Including these individuals in the profession would undoubtedly involve radical shifts in what it means to be 'a doctor'.

But this is never going to happen until doctors are given more effective ways of managing their anxieties. Doctors who are currently healthy and able-bodied can become unwell and disabled at any time. So in reality, the roles can be reversed, and the doctor – or somebody they love – can become the patient. This highly unwelcome thought has to be kept at bay if they are to cope with the psychological demands of treating patients. Currently the culture of medicine manages this potential anxiety by reifying the difference between doctors and patients as if they were separate species.

And sick or disabled doctors, whose very presence challenge this fundamental split, get pushed out of the profession.

6

Leaky Pipes

Tall, soberly dressed in dark colours, with no visible jewellery except a plain gold wedding band, Bridget didn't seek to mark herself out. Neither did she attempt to shove her success down your throat. Bridget wasn't the sort of person who needed you to know quite how extraordinary her achievements had been. But they *were* extraordinary; Bridget was one of the most gifted doctors I've encountered over the past twenty years.

Shortly after the birth of her second child Bridget contacted me. She wasn't sure whether or not she wanted to continue in her current job. Neurosurgery. Competition in the specialty is intense, and Bridget was one of a handful of women across the country who had obtained a much-coveted training position. But five years into her training programme, Bridget was having serious doubts about whether she wanted to be a neurosurgeon for the rest of her career.

In our first session, I asked Bridget why she had chosen medicine. She told me that becoming a doctor had been her 'default' option; her father was a surgeon, as was his father, and as she had excelled in all three sciences at school, studying medicine had always been a possibility. The problem, however, was that Bridget didn't only excel in the sciences at school – she was equally strong across the board. Had she wanted, she could have studied foreign languages or history or mathematics at university. And if that wasn't enough, she was also a gifted violinist and pianist.

At secondary school, her physics teacher (who had a PhD in the subject) recognised her talents and cautioned her against studying medicine. He suggested that she might find a subject such as theoretical physics more intellectually stimulating. But attracted to the breadth of medicine, and the wealth of opportunities a medical degree opened up, she ignored his advice.

As soon as she started her medical degree, the words of her teacher started to ring true. Whilst the volume of material to learn was enormous, there was little opportunity to study any topic in depth. Bridget found the work easy, but monotonous. In a genetics seminar she once asked a question which displayed such an advanced level of knowledge that the tutor assumed she had already completed a PhD. In reality she was only a second year medical student.

Things improved significantly when Bridget took a year out to complete an intercalated degree in neuroscience. She loved the interdisciplinary nature of the field, and her studie spanned neurology, philosophy and physiology. In addition gaining the top degree in the university, she won a natic prize for her research project. At this point she seriously considered leaving medicine and moving straight on to a PhD in neuroscience. But as is often the case, her family and her tutors encouraged her to return to her clinical training, assuring her that her options would be so much greater if she qualified as a doctor. With marked reluctance, she followed their advice.

Once Bridget had qualified as a doctor and completed the foundation programme, she had to decide on her specialty. With her stellar academic record, the breadth of her interests and the fact that she was highly dextrous, she had the pick of the bunch. In the end she opted for neurosurgery because it built on her earlier degree, required exquisite surgical dexterity, and would also allow her to contribute to interdisciplinary research into questions such as the origins of human consciousness. Given the competitiveness of the application process, Bridget didn't expect to be selected the first time she applied – but she was. The only problem was that the post she was offered was in the north of England, in a university town where she knew nobody. She accepted the offer, and headed north.

From the outset, her surgical supervisor made it clear that her face didn't fit. When other members of the team were present, he personified charm, but when nobody else was around, he constantly reminded Bridget that he hadn't wanted the position to go to a woman. Frequently he refused to let her join him in the operating theatre, so the only way that she could progress her neurosurgical skills was to approach other consultants and ask if she could 'scrub in' with them.

As Bridget pointed out, you can't become a surgeon just through studying textbooks in the library, in the same way that you can't learn how to ice-skate through watching videos of the Winter Olympics. For both you need to practise, practise and practise. With surgery, however, senior surgeons control access to hands-on experience in theatre. Of course this is necessary in terms of safeguarding the patient: the consultant has to assess whether a given trainee has the skills to carry out a particular surgical procedure. But controlling access in theatre isn't only about safeguarding patients – it's also about safeguarding a particular conception of who should become a surgeon.

Everything conspired to make Bridget feel unwelcome. She shared her office with the other trainees, all of whom were male. Sometimes, rather than going to the changing room, they would get undressed and change into theatre scrubs in the office. This made Bridget feel uncomfortable, but she didn't want to make a fuss so she never complained. At other times she had to push away colleagues' straying hands in theatre as they attempted to grope her breasts or pinch her bottom. When she attended academic conferences male colleagues phoned her hotel room at night, asking whether she would be willing to join them in bed.

On one occasion Bridget overheard a senior colleague say, 'Bridget is a naturally gifted surgeon.' But she was never given any positive feedback to her face. She stayed in the job because she kept on hoping that things would change. They didn't. So she was considerably relieved when th opportunity to do a PhD in London presented itself. She l the neurosurgical team and headed south to move into a research phase of her career.

Bridget's new research supervisor had recently been awarded a huge grant to carry out an international project across five research centres. With no prior experience of research administration, Bridget was left, with minimal supervision, to get the project off the ground. For the first year or so, although the workload was enormous, Bridget was relieved to escape the toxic harassment she had experienced in her earlier job. But the better she became at running the research project, the more trapped she started to feel.

'If Bridget got pregnant, the whole project would fall apart,' one of the senior consultants joked in a team meeting. Positive feedback – but not something that Bridget wanted to hear. The previous week she'd just had her first pregnancy confirmed. A month or so later, when she told her consultant, he was incandescent with rage. He would have to find somebody to take her place when she was on maternity leave.

The day after she gave birth to her first child, Bridget made the mistake of checking her emails. Her supervisor had sent her an academic paper that urgently needed revisions within the next couple of days. Bridget replied that she couldn't do the editing herself – she had a one-day-old baby. 'I'll write to the research funders and tell them about your lack of commitment,' was how he responded. 'This will ruin your research career,' he continued.

Shortly after her first pregnancy Bridget developed a rare ·toimmune disease. She returned to work after four months, ⁴ got the research project back on track – but at a considerable cost to her health. A year or so later she became pregnant again and, second time round, she was off for six months after the baby was born. Following her return to work after maternity leave, her health deteriorated significantly. Yet she continued working, determined to see the project through. None of her colleagues (many of whom were doctors) expressed any concern about her. That she was physically exhausted seemed to have escaped their notice. 'Can I have access to your database in case you die?' one of them quipped after Bridget had had a brief period of hospitalisation.

'Things got so bad that I felt that I couldn't be a neurosurgeon *and* a wife *and* a mother,' Bridget told me. 'It was killing me, and ruining my family. I didn't think it was worth it.'

Eventually Bridget met somebody at a conference who worked for a biotechnology start-up. They were looking for a clinician with a background in neuroscience, and asked her to apply. After the interview they were so keen to snap her up that they kept the job open for six months to allow her to finish her PhD.

'Would it have been different if you hadn't had children?' I asked. 'Might you still be training as a neurosurgeon?'

Bridget said she had allowed herself to leave *because* of the children. Despite the toll that neurosurgery training was taking on her own health, it was the impact on the children that ultimately proved the decisive factor.

'In my old job I spent every second of the day doing things, but even then there wasn't enough time for my work and my family. I was constantly exhausted. If I'd loved the wor' I would have got two nannies and enough help to mud through. But ultimately I decided I didn't love the work enough to go down that route.'

I asked Bridget what needs to change in order for women like her to survive in a specialty like neurosurgery. I anticipated that she would say something about greater sharing of family responsibilities within the home, or more effective sanctions against sexist bullying, or academic centres having more realistic expectations of the demands they can place on women with young children. But, being Bridget, she came up with something much more interesting:

'We need to broaden our concept of who a surgeon is,' she said, 'so that it includes women who have different approaches to work.'

'What do you mean?'

'In both the operating theatre and the lab, I was made to feel that I didn't fit in – that I didn't belong. Prior to my surgical training, I was complimented on how I communicated with patients as well as with colleagues. Once I started surgery, nurses and other health professionals said the same. "We need more surgeons like you," they said. But the surgical consultants told me that I wasn't sufficiently "surgeon like" – despite the fact that there was never any criticism of my clinical skills in theatre. People wanted me to be somebody else. Somebody who I wasn't.'

'What did people say when you left?' I asked.

'Nothing. There was no exit interview. No one bothered to get in touch. I was erased from history.'

Despite being appointed, against ferocious competition, to ̶e of the most prestigious training programmes in the UK, ̶ody was interested in why Bridget left.

Recently I met up with Bridget, three months after she had started her new job. By most people's standards she was working extremely hard; in addition to her demanding new role she had a train commute of two hours each way. But she used the commuting time for extra reading (she's started an online Master's in computational neuroscience) as well as sorting out family stuff.

'My opinion is valued,' she said. 'People are interested in what I have to say. For the first time in years, I can be myself.'

*

In 1988 Isobel Allen published a study of women doctors. Commissioned by the Department of Health, the study was based on face-to-face interviews with doctors (both male and female) who had graduated in 1966, 1976 and 1981. 'Women were conspicuous by their absence' in the higher surgical grades, Allen noted. Roll the clock forward to 2009 and the National Working Group on Women in Medicine, also commissioned by the Department of Health, concluded that 'surgery is an area of particular concern, given the relatively low percentage of women in such a large specialty'. This report then goes on to make nine recommendations – most of which are entirely predictable (improved access to mentoring, career advice, part-time working, flexible training, adequate childcare). These recommendations sound positive, but you couldn't say they were forward thinking. Identical suggestions had been made twenty years earlier in Isobel Allen's report.

In fact many of these recommendations have been doing the rounds for thirty or forty years. Same old, same old, same c

But we are *still* in a position where a study published in the *British Medical Journal* in 2016 reported that

> Trainees described negative attitudes from seniors towards pregnancy and maternity/paternity leave, and towards trainees – especially women – who wanted to work less than full time . . . Negative attitudes were most often reported to be from senior male doctors and/or in surgical specialties.

It's hard to escape the conclusion that all these government reports and academic papers and working groups are somehow missing the point. To use a medical analogy, if somebody is infected by the rubella virus, they may have a range of symptoms such as a red rash, fever, or swollen lymph nodes. You can treat the symptoms once somebody is infected (give paracetamol, for instance) and it will help the individual patient. But prescribing paracetamol isn't going to reduce the incidence of rubella in the population. For that you have to tackle the underlying cause – the rubella virus – through population-based immunisation programmes.

And it's the same with treating the problem of women in surgery. The lack of role models and mentors, the prejudice against women working part-time, the bullying and sexual harassment are symptoms. They are not the end of the story. Treating the problem at this level is like dishing out paracetamol to patients with rubella. It will probably help a few women surgeons here and there, but to solve the problem you need to deal with the underlying cause – the professional culture of surgery – that, even in the second decade of the twenty-first century, remains hostile to women.

If you want to understand a virus, ask a virologist. If you want to know how viral infections spread throughout a population, ask an epidemiologist. And if you want to know how the professional culture of surgery damages women's careers you need to ask somebody who studies cultures – a social anthropologist or sociologist. It's from their observations of surgery in action that answers can be found.

Joan Cassell, a social anthropologist, studied the culture of surgery. She did more than interview female surgeons however – she also scrubbed in and went into operating theatres. In total she observed thirty-three women surgeons over a three-year period. And what did she find? Not simply that the culture of surgery is essentially masculine, but that surgical culture *embodies* masculinity. In other words, this masculinity is expressed through the *body* of the surgeon. To understand the difficulties that women face in terms of 'sexism' is too abstract, Cassell argues. Too disembodied, in fact. Only by taking account of the embodied nature of surgical practice can you explain the visceral response that female surgeons such as Bridget can encounter – a response that tells them that they are the wrong body in the wrong place.

Surgery is not the only occupation that embodies masculinity. Cassell mentions test-piloting and racing-car driving, grouping them together as 'death-haunted' pursuits. She doesn't mention the military – but I would certainly add it to the list. It was not until December 2015 that women in the US military were allowed to serve in all front-line combat positions; the UK followed suit the following year, opening up front-line infantry and tank positions to female soldiers. If your line of work (racing-car driver, tank commander, surgeon) embodies what it means to be pre-eminently male in a particular culture, then the presence of a woman will be resisted.

From my own observations in theatre, I was often struck by how extraordinary it was that one person (the surgeon) cuts into the body of another (the patient). Cassell graphically describes this physical nature of surgery: 'During an operation the body of the surgeon makes brutal contact with the body of the patient, piercing the envelope of skin, assaulting the flesh, violating body integrity.'

Of course this 'brutal contact' is inflicted for the patient's benefit (as opposed to such contact by soldiers, where the aim is to benefit one's country by wounding or killing the enemy). Surgical work (like front-line combat) embodies our cultural view of the characteristics of masculinity – decisiveness, the ability to take command, physical strength.

This notion that surgery embodies masculinity also explains why female surgeons are treated with particular hostility during pregnancy. Cassell describes one female resident who needed bed rest towards the end of her pregnancy and who was threatened by her Chief Resident, who told her that her salary would be cut. This resident remonstrated with the Chief, pointing out that she had accumulated vacation and sick leave and that anyway the amount of time she was having away from the operating theatre was no greater than the amount taken by military doctors who were training alongside her. As Cassell comments:

Taking time off for war is such supremely surgical behaviour that it goes almost unnoticed: the iron surgeon is by definition a warrior who engages in hand-to-hand combat with disease and death. Taking time off for pregnancy, on the other hand, is intensely unsurgical: being pregnant and having a baby designates one's body as that of a patient or a wife.

Through painstaking observations, Cassell witnessed how dramatic surgical 'saves' were valorised over compassionate, clinically informed surgical care. And even when women surgeons *did* perform dramatic surgical interventions, the male audience assumed that something must have been done wrong. As an example, one female resident told Cassell about a technically demanding surgical procedure she had carried out that had undoubtedly saved the patient's life. This resident described the case in the weekly M & M (morbidity and mortality) meeting – a forum where adverse or exceptional outcomes get discussed by the whole surgical team. Despite the success of the surgery, she was criticised for tiny details, and her achievement was entirely overlooked. This was in sharp contrast to the response the following week to a male resident, who was widely praised for his role in a far simpler case. In the view of the female resident: 'If I reported at M & M that I had resurrected Lazarus, they would ask me why I'd waited four days.'

Unsurprisingly, Cassell concludes that female surgeons are in a 'double bind'. If they're not exceptional they probably won't make it through their training. If they are exceptional they will be 'the nail that sticks out and gets hammered in'.

*

I couldn't stop thinking how, twenty years after Cassell had carried out her observational research, all the key themes emerged from Bridget's story: the way in which she was made to feel that she didn't belong in the operating theatre; the hostility to her pregnancy; how her supervisors overlooked her undoubted surgical competence and instead criticised her compassionate patient care – to list just a few examples.

Cassell and other authors have shown that even the most exceptional female doctors may struggle against the power of a medical (and particularly surgical) establishment that remains deeply hostile to them. In terms of her achievements, Bridget was exceptional, but sadly in terms of her experiences, she was not. A study published in the *American Journal of Surgery* in 2016 reached the following conclusion:

> Over half the women in our study stated they felt they had been discriminated against, based on their gender. Furthermore, the results showed that the perception of gender discrimination seemed to increase as they moved up through the ranks of medical student, to resident, and to staff surgeon.

Another study, published in 2016 in the *British Medical Journal*, reported the following responses from trainee female surgeons:

> The surgical environment is a male bastion, whether or not we like to acknowledge it. If it's changed, it's slowly but it's still very, very male dominated. So maternity leave is a dirty word . . . I had this very negative reaction from

my consultant at the time in the unit when I told them I was pregnant. Very negative. He chastised me for it . . . It was soul destroying.

I've had people say to me, 'You're either a woman or a neurosurgeon, you can't be both.'

And according to Jyoti Shah, a consultant urological surgeon in the UK, female surgeons still encounter comments about menstruation in the operating theatre. If they speak out, male colleagues might enquire 'Is it the time of the month?'

Whether the remarks are about periods or pregnancy, their frequency suggests that women are still being told, in one way or another, that they have the wrong body to train as a surgeon.

*

Of course it was far far worse for the female medical pioneers. In 1863 Elizabeth Garrett Anderson wrote to the Aberdeen Medical School, requesting permission to attend anatomy classes. This is the response she received:

I have so strong a conviction that the entrance of ladies into dissecting-rooms and anatomical theatres is so undesirable in every respect, and highly unbecoming that I could not do anything to promote your end . . . It is indeed necessary for the purpose of Surgery and Medicine that these matters should be studied, but fortunately it is not necessary that fair ladies should be brought into contact with such foul scenes . . . Ladies would make bad doctors at the best, and they do so

many things excellently, that I for one should be sorry to *see
them trying to do this one.*

Undeterred, Garrett Anderson followed other routes, and eventually found her way on to the medical register. Together with
Sophia Jex-Blake, she later founded the London School of
Medicine for Women in 1874. Three years later, female medical
students were able to gain access to clinical experience through
the London Free Hospital, and two years after that, an Act of
Parliament granted relevant institutions the authority to let
women qualify as doctors.

American women faced similar obstacles. The influential
Canadian physician William Osler, first Professor of Medicine
at the newly founded Johns Hopkins Medical School in
Baltimore and later Regius Professor of Medicine at Oxford
University, opposed opening up the profession to women. Osler
argued that the professional demeanour of the doctor should
be characterised by equanimity – the capacity to remain cool,
calm and collected in all situations. According to Osler, women
lacked this essential capacity, and thus would never make good
doctors. In the 1890s Osler joked with his (male) students that
'humankind might be divided into three categories – men,
women and women physicians'. A light-hearted quip perhaps,
but giving voice to a similar sentiment to the writer from
Aberdeen Medical School: real women don't become doctors.

Yet women continued to demand access to the medical
profession – despite facing considerable obstacles. In the UK
opportunities for women expanded during the First World War,
but most of the places made available during this period were

subsequently withdrawn after the war. In 1921 women still made up only 5.4% of the total medical workforce. By the end of the Second World War, 25% of medical students were female, although their student numbers were decreased after the war as ex-servicemen returned to claim university places. One step forward, one step back. In 1962, just over 20% of UK medical students were women, but twenty years later the proportion had risen to 45.3%. By 1992, female students outnumbered their male colleagues, and that is the way it has stayed ever since. Latest figures for the UK show that 55% of medical students are women.

The feminisation of the US medical workforce has consistently lagged behind. Whilst women were admitted to Oxford Medical School from 1916, they were denied this option at Harvard and Yale until after the Second World War. In fact, it was only after a significant change in legislation in 1972 (Title IX of the Education Amendments) that discriminatory admissions policies were outlawed in institutions receiving federal funds. As a result, between 1970 and 1980, the proportion of female medical students more than doubled, from 12.3 to 28%. And the latest figures, for 2016 entry, indicate that for the first time ever, parity has almost been achieved: 49.8% women compared to 50.2% men. Almost, but not quite.

Yet these figures on access to the profession can be deceptive. Underneath a thin veneer of equity lie significant differences in the career trajectories of male and female doctors. This becomes clear when one looks at the particular specialties that women doctors end up pursuing.

*

Olivia, a married doctor with three young children, came to see me because she felt she had ended up in the wrong specialty. In our first session she told me that she had volunteered in an orphanage in India before starting medical school, and the country had got under her skin. Her love of the country pulled her back during her elective period in medical school, when she returned to work in the hospital attached to the orphanage, and she returned again once she qualified. From the time of her elective, when she had encountered patients suffering from a wide range of infections, Olivia decided that infectious diseases was the specialty for her. She loved the fact that some of the conditions were extremely rare and tricky to diagnose; the specialty demanded 'detective work'. She also found it hugely satisfying that many patients with an infectious disease could make remarkable recoveries once the disease had been correctly diagnosed and treated. And she sensed that the specialty attracted kindred spirits – people like her, who were committed to working in the developing world.

But in the UK, infectious diseases is a highly competitive specialty. It's difficult to get a place on a training scheme and, as with other competitive specialties, studying for a PhD, on top of completing the clinical aspects of training, has become the norm. To make matters worse, whereas in the past infectious disease trainees would often have had a reasonably light out-of-hours schedule, nowadays this has all changed. The shift isn't due to pedagogical demands; you can learn how to be a first-class infectious disease specialist without staffing the hospital at night or at weekends. Instead, it is entirely due to staff shortages.

Olivia didn't want to study for a PhD alongside her clinical work. She didn't want to have to worry about churning out publications or meeting funding application deadlines and she didn't want to work lots of evenings and weekends. With three children, she decided that training in the specialty would be unmanageable, so after a lot of soul searching, she opted instead for general practice.

As soon as she started working as a GP she realised she had made a dreadful mistake. Olivia enjoyed treating very sick patients whom she could make better. Quickly. She liked diagnostic challenges, with clear definable outcomes. Now if patients presented with serious, puzzling symptoms she referred them to hospital specialists. From her point of view, it was her hospital colleagues who were doing all the detective work, and having all the fun.

There's also evidence that patients bring different problems to male and female GPs. Women GPs see a higher proportion of female-specific and psychosocial problems. In contrast, male GPs are more frequently consulted about musculoskeletal and respiratory problems, as well as male genital problems. Not surprisingly, given that patients are more likely to consult female GPs about complex psychosocial issues, they tend to have a significantly higher proportion of lengthy consultations than their male GP colleagues. It wasn't that Olivia was uncaring – she just liked to be presented with well-defined clinical problems that could be quickly cured. Long-term depression, or anxiety, or alcoholism, coupled with a whole host of social and financial difficulties, don't fall into this category. But these were th sorts of patients who came knocking on Olivia's surgery door asking for help.

Olivia was not alone in choosing general practice over a hospital specialty in order to give priority to her family life. A 2015 study asked over 15,000 doctors in the UK about the factors that had influenced their specialty choices. GPs were much more likely to attribute their decision to 'wanting a career with acceptable working hours' and 'wanting a career that fits in with my domestic situation' than doctors in any other specialty. This isn't necessarily a problem, and many GPs enjoy their work enormously. But doctors who select their specialty on the basis of a shorter working day, or less time on call, are in effect choosing their job because it gives them more time *not* doing the job. This is just like teachers who go into the profession solely because of the long holidays. Of course evenings, weekends and holidays are all crucially important for one's well-being. In the longer run, however, people in demanding professions such as teaching or medicine also need to derive satisfaction from the time they spend *at* work, rather than staying in their jobs because it allows them more time to be away from work.

Olivia knew nothing about general practice before she chose it as her lifelong specialty. From our discussions, she has come to the conclusion that she is better suited to hospital medicine. She has also accepted that the research demands of infectious disease, coupled with the hours of work, mean that it probably wouldn't work for her either. But she is exploring whether a specialty such as sexual medicine might be a good alternative. This specialty includes a lot of infectious diseases work (treating patients suffering from sexually transmitted infections), is largely outpatient based, and would also allow her to do stints working in HIV clinics in India. That's the good news. The bad news is that leaving general practice and qualifying as a consultant will require at least four more years of full-time training – and she might find it difficult to get accepted on to a scheme in the part of the country where she currently lives with her husband and three young children. Her problems are not yet over.

*

As many female doctors choose general practice because of the flexibility it offers, women are over-represented amongst GPs, and under-represented amongst hospital consultants. Two hospital specialties, however, buck this trend and have a majority of female consultants. Just two. Not surprisingly these two specialties are obstetrics/gynaecology and paedi-atrics; women doctors flourish, as long as they are dealing with 'womanly' problems such as pregnancy, childbirth and children.

And the hospital specialty with the lowest proportion of female consultants? Surgery. In 2016 just 12% of surgical consultants were women. This difference can't be explained away in terms of women not being interested in or good at surgical procedures, as obstetrics/gynaecology could techni-cally be defined as a surgical specialty. And with acute obstet-rics, unlike every other surgical specialty, the surgeon has to safeguard the well-being of two patients (mother and baby) rather than just one. Yet in the UK, the proportion of female consultants in obstetrics/gynaecology is over four times greater (51%) than the proportion of female consultants in other surgical specialties.

Women doctors don't only cluster in different specialties; they are also much more likely to work part-time. So for example, a 2016 survey of over 10,000 doctors in the UK found that whilst 42% of women worked part-time, the comparable figure amongst men was 7%. The proportion of part-time medics was also skewed by specialty; amongst female GPs, 40% worked part-time whilst amongst female surgeons, the figure was 10%. Women in surgical specialties are still very much in the minority – and when they do choose these specialties, they are highly unlikely to work part-time. This study also showed clearly that the critical factor was children. In fact female doctors without children were no more likely to work part-time than male doctors with, or without, children.

Family considerations also impact on the proportion of female doctors choosing to go down an academic clinical pathway. Doctors who choose this type of career have to complete the same demanding clinical training but *on top of* *this* have to carry out research, write academic papers and complete complex applications for continued research funding. Given that doctors in the US have clinical schedules of eighty hours per week, it's clear why opting for a chunky additional set of tasks might put women off – particularly if they go home to equally chunky domestic responsibilities. Even in the UK, where working hours are constrained by the European Working ¯ime Directive and integrated academic training pathways have been devised, a significant gender imbalance remains in academic medicine – particularly at senior levels.

As in so many other professions, within medicine women are paid less than their male counterparts. In part this discrepancy is due to the fact that across the consultant workforce as a whole women consultants tend to be younger, are more likely to have had career breaks, and are less likely to hold high-profile administrative or research posts. These factors account for about 60% of the pay gap between male and female consultants. The remaining 40% is caused by the fact that women get different financial rewards for the *same* achievements. For example, a premium for being a professor adds 22% to a man's salary, but only 8% to a woman's. Men who have been in their consultant post for ten years earn 34% more than a recently appointed consultant, yet for women this difference is only 13%. And it's not just in the UK; similar salary discrepancies between male and female doctors doing exactly the same work have been reported in the US.

As Sir Liam Donaldson, the then UK Chief Medical Officer, wrote in 2009: 'the problem is not access to medical school, but rather how we ensure that the female medical workforce is able to fulfil its potential once in employment'. The step on the bottom rung of the medical ladder may be equally accessible to men and women. But it's a long ladder. Once women climb up the first few steps, the notion of gender parity looks less convincing. The particular pathway chosen, how high up someone is able to climb, and even the amount they will get paid for their labours differ between the two sexes.

*

An email pings into my inbox:

Dear Caroline

I went into medicine as a postgraduate so unlike my colleagues I am a little older and am married with two wee girls. At this point my priorities lie far less with my career progression and much more with preserving a happy family life . . . I feel that I have hit a junction in my medical career with some stark choices to make and I feel a lot of responsibility in making this choice – I just want to get it right. I've begun to suffer from insomnia which is new for me and though I don't lie awake ruminating nor feel low in mood I know that this is a sign that I cannot plough ahead as I have been.

I get emails like this all the time and many of the doctors who come to see me bring stories about the impossibility of balancing work and family life. Typically these stories are told by women, but sometimes (as with the email above) it's men who agonise about the toll that their medical work is having on their children.

Specialty training in the UK can last for more than ten years after leaving medical school. That's ten years of full-time work. Or twenty years, if you are working part-time. During this period you will change job, with little choice as to where you get sent, every six to twelve months. As one doctor put it – 'the system moves you around like a piece of equipment rather than a person'. And if the constant moving isn't bad enough, some of these jobs may involve a considerable commute. From a logistical point of view, trying to arrange childcare can be a nightmare. But that's not all.

With each move you will need to get to know new colleagues and work in different hospitals, so you quickly have to learn how things are done in your new place of work. For the first few years there is the relentless pressure of postgraduate exams, and throughout the whole of your training you are constantly being assessed by your seniors. Now some specialties have introduced exit exams as well, at the end of training. And on top of all of this, there is an ever-increasing load of extraneous tasks that every doctor needs to complete each year in order to get through their annual review and be allowed to progress to the next step of training. Imagine trying to do all of this stuff to keep one's training on track, for ten to twenty years *alongside* looking after one's family.

The bottom line is that medicine is not an accommodating profession when it comes to supporting doctors with childcare (or indeed any other caring) responsibilities. Some of this lack of accommodation comes with the territory; sick patients need care twenty-four hours a day. Typically an accountancy or architecture problem can wait till the following morning. Acutely unwell patients cannot. But it's not only the clinical needs of patients that make medicine a challenging career choice for women. The profession as a whole has not yet fully adapted to a feminised workforce, many of whom are attempting to combine their medical training with looking after a family for years and years on end.

The responses to a survey of women doctors carried out by the BMA in 2009 give a good sense of the career challenges that these individuals face:

'I was offered but had to turn down a clinical senior lecturer post because I cannot work as few hours as I need to and the responsibilities are too great to juggle with new motherhood.'

'A female colleague who was childless was promoted over my head despite much lower experience, but I applied for promotion through an appeal process and got it.'

'Senior female staff exist in our organisation but they do not have children and take the view that we should be "flexible" and prepared to relocate if necessary.'

'Being part-time, still regarded as inferior to full-time male colleagues.'

'I had to wait 8 years for a part-time consultant post.'

'It is still a man's world – especially at the top.'

In the US, it's even worse. Part-time work may hamper one's career prospects, but in the UK the official guidance states that all doctors can apply for flexible training, and that every application will be treated 'positively'. In contrast, in America, maternity leave following the birth of a child is far shorter (twelve weeks as opposed to six months), and opportunities for training part-time are often scarce. Studies are replete with horror stories that women faced when they attempted to continue training with a young family:

When at age 37, I delivered my firstborn 1 week to the day after beginning a fellowship in high-risk pregnancy, I was devastated to have him admitted to the neonatal intensive care unit. On my way out the door, I ran into the senior fellow who said to me, 'Too bad about what happened. When can I put you back on the call schedule?'

With all these difficulties, it's hardly surprising that many women, and some men too, leave hospital medicine to work as a GP. It's not that this is an easy option. Far from it. But with general practice in the UK or primary care options in the US, the postgraduate training is shorter than in hospital specialties, part-time schedules can be more easily accommodated, and there are few or no compulsory night shifts. In both the UK and the US there are also shortages of primary care physicians, so finding a training scheme and later a job in the right part of the country tends to be easier. Yet sometimes these doctors, like Olivia, become haunted by the path not taken. They constantly ask themselves whether things would have been better if they had followed their heart and tried to complete their training in a hospital specialty.

*

Other women make different choices; they decide to slog it out through their hospital training in order to qualify in their chosen specialty – even if their training extends well over a decade. But then, like Sally, they can encounter different problems.

Sally came to see me when she was close to finishing her training in cardiology. Except that she wasn't *really* close; as she was training part-time, she was still two to three years away from completion. Her training had dragged on and on. First of all, she had taken a few years after leaving medical school, rotating through different specialties before she finally decided on cardiology. Then she had four children – the last of whom was born prematurely, and needed to be hospitalised for the first month of his life. Following each pregnancy she had taken a year's maternity leave. In addition, as competition for cardiology consultant posts is intense, she had been advised to complete a PhD on top of her clinical training. Sally was struggling to motivate herself to write up her thesis, and began the first session by telling me that she felt her career had hit a brick wall.

When I asked Sally about her parents' careers she told me that her father had been a physician and her mother had given up her career on starting a family. She remembered that, as a child, she'd always thought her father's work sounded tremendously exciting, and from an early age she decided she wanted to train as a doctor. But Sally also talked about how pleased she had been each day when she came home from school to find her mother waiting for her, with home-made biscuits and cake. It was almost as if Sally was being pulled in opposite directions – wanting to be the clever, academic doctor (like her father) as well as a devoted mother who was there at the end of each day for her children. Not an easy tension to reconcile.

What shocked me most, however, about Sally's story was the totally inadequate preparation for her returning to treat acutely unwell patients. When Sally came to see me, it was six years since she had been responsible for treating patients whose life was in the balance. This period away from acute practice stacked up because of the four maternity leaves and a number of years in a research lab. When she raised her concerns with her clinical supervisor – what did he suggest? A one-day refresher course?

So Sally had to kick and scream, and demand a more appropriate schedule for her return to work. She didn't do this to make trouble, or to ask for special concessions. Instead, she refused to go back on to the on-call register as soon as she started her new job, because she knew she wasn't safe. She wanted to have a supervised refresher period. This request was entirely in accordance with the GMC guidance that as a doctor you have to 'recognise and work within the limits of your competence'. But her senior colleagues were none too pleased and gave her a negative report in her training record, for the first time ever.

Over the years I have encountered a number of doctors like Sally who, for one reason or another, have spent considerable periods of time away from acutely sick patients. And frequently (although not invariably) the provision made for their induction back into acute medicine is woefully inadequate. The training system as a whole hasn't yet adapted to the reality of repeated maternity leaves coupled with returning to part-time clinical work interspersed with periods doing research. There's a fundamental mismatch between the educational needs of the doctor and the return-to-practice support provided by the hospitals.

*

On the face of it, things might seem easier for female hospital doctors who don't have partners or children: they are certainly more likely to work full-time. But sometimes these doctors feel that they have paid too high a price to complete their training in a hospital specialty. I also wonder whether this problem isn't particularly acute with international medical graduates (IMGs). It can take IMGs a number of years before they obtain a place on a training scheme and in the intervening period, they often take short-term six-month posts all over the country. It's difficult to build up a solid social network if you move around like this, yet these are the years when people are most likely to be meeting a future partner. Even when these doctors finally get a training place on top of their busy medical job there will be exams to pass (sometimes in a second language) as well as building up skills in research, clinical audit and teaching. Some of these additional tasks may be less familiar to doctors who trained outside the UK so again they can be particularly time-consuming for IMGs. 'I was entirely focused on completing my training and getting a job as a consultant,' was what one doctor said to me. And this focus can have a detrimental impact on a doctor's life outside work.

In my sessions with doctors I often ask them about things that they have done at work which they are particularly proud of. The answers to this question never cease to amaze me; arranging a wedding for a terminally ill young man in a hospice; setting up a falls service for older patients that won a national award; improving the transition from paediatric to adult services for adolescent patients with sickle cell anaemia. But when I alter the question and ask doctors for things they have done *outside* of work which have made them proud, quite frequently they remain silent. Sometimes the sense of regret can be palpable. Little wonder then that a respondent in another study of female doctors concluded that 'medicine is one big career of loss'.

*

'Ladies would make bad doctors, at the best,' Elizabeth Garrett Anderson was told, when she wanted to attend the anatomy lectures at Aberdeen Medical School back in 1863. I wonder what the writer of that letter would make of the findings of a study published in February 2017 in the *Journal of the American Medical Association*. The study conducted by a group of researchers at Harvard School of Public Health analysed thirty-day mortality and readmission rates of over a million patients aged sixty-five years and older, hospitalised with a medical condition between 2011 and 2014. And what did they find? That patients treated by female physicians had lower thirty-day mortality rates, and lower readmission rates. These differences persisted across eight common medical conditions and were not found to be dependent upon the patients' severity of illness. In a nutshell, sick older patients did better if the doctor who admitted them to hospital was a woman.

An editorial about the study, in the same issue of the journal, suggested that the improved outcomes for patients treated by female physicians may be because women are more likely to stick to clinical guidelines, or because they communicate more effectively with patients and tend to have longer consultations than their male colleagues. At this point the precise mechanism causing the difference in clinical outcome remains unclear. But it would be hard to disagree with the conclusion reached by Professor Jane Dacre, a former president of the Royal College of Physicians of London, that medicine is 'richer' for diversity in its workforce.

The old arguments against doctors working part-time don't stack up either. Not only is there evidence that doctors who work less than full-time are less stressed and more satisfied at work, but in future it seems likely that the proportion of male doctors choosing this option will increase. As a group of researchers from Oxford University concluded in a 2016 paper, medicine needs to establish legitimate career paths that enable doctors of *both* sexes to train and work part-time.

Another senior female clinician, Professor Fiona Karet Frankl based in Cambridge, wrote recently about her dismay on learning that a female medical student had been advised by a senior male surgeon not to choose a career in surgery – 'Surely you will want to have a family?' the surgeon asked. Subsequently, Karet Frankl heard almost identical stories from colleagues in several other medical schools.

'When I started medical school in 1980, 52% of my class was female but some 35 years later, only 13% of my professorial cohort is,' Karet Frankl wrote. Then she went on to say, 'we speak of a "leaky" pipeline, but further discussion often focuses on the water rather than the pipe'.

In my discussions with female doctors, I've seen how they 'leak out' of the hospital medicine pipeline into part-time community-based roles. Or they leak out of medicine entirely. There's no getting round the fact that the first decade of a medical career coincides with the time when a woman is most likely to be getting married and wanting to start a family. Part-time work is more readily accessible in the UK, which eases the pressure a bit, but it extends training, sometimes for years and years on end.

My friend's daughter, Sophie, who started an obstetrics and gynaecology residency in the US in 2016, was offered the option to freeze her eggs, by some of the residency training programmes to which she applied. But isn't there something perverse about an obstetrics and gynaecology programme enticing residents with the offer of egg freezing when the gynaecologists and obstetricians working on the programme know that the rate of conception with frozen eggs is lower than making babies the old-fashioned way?

And can't we find better ways to allow brilliant doctors like Bridget to continue working in the profession? Ways that would allow her to feel that she fitted into the surgical team and had something of value to contribute.

7

Risky Business

I once went to see the dean of one of the London medical schools. The purpose of the meeting was to review whether his medical school could be doing more to help prepare students for the specialty choice decisions they would have to make a year or so after graduation. In the course of the discussion the dean told me that his institution had too many Asian girls who weren't actually interested in becoming doctors, but were only interested in marriage.

I have little doubt that if Professor *only-interested-in-marriage* met a client of mine called Rahma he would find confirmation of his views about female, Asian medical students. Rahma, who grew up in London, was the only child of older parents. She had been brought up to be respectful of her elders and quietly mannered with people she didn't know well. All of her friends at school and at her sixth form college came from similar backgrounds within the UK Pakistani community.

From the beginning of medical school, Rahma realised that she was different from many of the students she encountered and she told me that she felt much less confident than many of her peers. She hadn't travelled the world in her gap year – indeed she had never contemplated doing so because her family couldn't afford that sort of luxury. And she didn't share the extracurricular accomplishments of many of her privately educated fellow students, be these in music, sport, debating, or whatever. Fencing, rowing, or playing the harp weren't on offer to students in the school and sixth form college she had attended.

'Being self-assured goes a long way in medicine,' Rahma told me. And it's true. Unlike, say, a degree in history or economics, which will consist largely of lectures, seminars and private study, at medical school students' knowledge and skills are constantly exposed to senior clinicians and to patients, as part of their clinical training. On a ward round, when Rahma was with a group of students at the bedside of a patient, she wouldn't be the first to answer the consultant's questions. Neither did she rush to ask the consultant any questions that she had; she was wary of senior medics, and hesitant to initiate conversation. But when consultants like Professor *only-interested-in-marriage* encountered students like Rahma, they didn't see an incredibly bright but shy young woman, who needed encouragement. What they saw was somebody who wasn't interested in becoming a doctor. In other words, their reading of the situation confirmed their initial stereotype.

So what happens next?

Teaching is a reciprocal activity. The consultant clocks the shy Asian girl who doesn't volunteer questions or answers, and directs his next instruction (listen to the patient's heart and tell me what you hear) to somebody else. Actually Rahma was confident that she knew the different heart sounds and would have liked to be asked. Disappointed that she wasn't given the opportunity, she retreats further into her shell, which provides additional confirmation to the consultant that students like Rahma aren't committed to the profession.

'I was too shy and hesitant to get noticed,' Rahma told me. 'Maybe my interest in medicine didn't show.' Throughout her six years at medical school there were hundreds of daily encounters where she was misread; encounters which meant that opportunities for building up her confidence or furthering her learning were missed. Rahma had a particular interest in dermatology and chose one of her optional modules in this specialty. But she couldn't convey her passion to the module supervisor; he didn't respond to her emails, and she missed out on the opportunity to get some research experience that would have greatly enhanced her CV later on in her career.

'What am I not doing, that I'm not getting the opportunity to take part in research?' Rahma asked herself. Rather than blaming her supervisors, she began to believe that she must be lacking in some way, which led to yet more erosion of confidence. And on it went to the point that although she passed her medical school finals with no difficulty whatsoever, she was completely overwhelmed when she started her first job as a junior hospital doctor. Which is when she first came to see me.

*

'Siblings never have the same parents,' a psychologist colleague once remarked. What she meant by this puzzling statement is that, with the exception of twins, each additional sibling will arrive when the parents are at a different stage in their marriage, or career, or family life. For example, an older child might have been born at a time of marital stability whilst a later child arrives when the marriage is in difficulty. And each child will have their own personality and physical appearance, reminding parents of other relatives – perhaps a brother whom the father looked up to, or a sister with whom he always competed. This then sets up a pattern of interaction, gathering momentum as it plays out over time. When one looks in detail at how parents respond to their different children, the notion that siblings don't share the same parents starts to make sense.

It's the same with education. Students from different ethnicities – even if they grew up in the UK, and sit in the same lecture theatre at medical school – don't have the same day-to-day educational experiences. Professor *only-interested-in marriage* wasn't alone in his views about Asian students and there is good evidence that negative stereotypes are common. In a paper published in the *British Medical Journal* in 2008 psychologist Kath Woolf described numerous examples of negative stereotypes of Asian students perpetuated by both students and clinical teachers:

'Some of these sweet little Asian girlies are very hard to get through to. I'm quite a physically biggish sort of chap, maybe that's another factor. I'm older, obviously that's a factor. I'm male. I'm . . . they don't communicate terribly well.' (Teacher, male consultant, white)

'They came over in the sixties when Idi Amin kicked them out, they're very keen on their children achieving excellent attributes. So their children bloody well have to work, there's a work ethic at home, um, and they get three A grades at A level so the authorities let them in because they think three As at A level's a good thing, which I think is bonkers.' (Teacher, male consultant, white)

'There's a stigma of sort of ethnic families wanting their children to do best and then there's the whole doctor, lawyer, you know, get the upper, upper rank jobs or whatever they're called and so I suppose if they're thinking "oh bollocks, I've got to choose between three jobs, I'll choose the doctor then."' (Student, male, white)

If clinical teachers and students openly express these views to a bright-eyed and bushy-tailed research psychologist who has come to interview them, what do they say when the researcher isn't there? Little wonder then that the paper concluded:

Teachers of clinical medical students, and the students themselves, have strong perceptions about 'typical' Asian students, and there is a systematic mismatch between these perceptions and the (equally strong) perception of what makes a 'good' clinical student. These findings are consistent with the hypothesis that negative stereotypes of Asian medical students exist.

*

A recent incident at Cardiff Medical School provides further evidence of the widespread nature of negative stereotyping amongst medical students. In 2016 a complaint was made by a group of black students at the medical school following the performance of a student revue. Events of this type happen in many medical schools, and provide an opportunity for students to make fun of teaching staff under the guise of raising money for a suitable charity. At Cardiff, one of the lecturers who was lampooned was black. And how was he portrayed? By a white student with a blacked-up face, wearing an over-sized dildo. The stereotype of the over-sexualised black man played out for all to enjoy.

When a group of BME (black and minority ethnic) students complained, they were told by those who participated in the revue that there had been a warning at the beginning of the show about the nature of the content, and they should have left, if they felt sensitive about race. (I wouldn't want to be treated by these particular revue participants when they grow up and become doctors.)

Following the complaint and the subsequent investigation by the medical school, the student body as a whole became irreparably divided. The complainants reported that they were ostracised, and as a consequence some of them decided to continue their medical training elsewhere. Another group of fifth year medical students started a Facebook petition to let the dean know that there was nothing wrong in the revue, and that they stood in solidarity with their colleagues who had taken part. And some of the students involved in the revue never understood why the content had been criticised in the first place.

In the end an independent review panel had to be drafted in, headed up by Dinesh Bhugra, Professor of Mental Health and Diversity at the Institute of Psychiatry in London. Not surprisingly, in their report the independent panel made recommendations that went far beyond overseeing the content of the student revue: complaints procedures; support for staff; training in diversity and equality; the medical school curriculum and mentoring were some of the issues raised. Because incidents like this are never merely about a small group of students.

*

'The hardest attitude to change is the one you don't know you have,' wrote John Dovidio, a professor in the Department of Psychology at Yale University.

I'm not sure whether Professor *only-interested-in-marriage* or the Cardiff medical students were aware of holding racist attitudes. But I am sure that each and every one of us holds unconscious beliefs about people whom we perceive to be different from ourselves. These beliefs may be outside our conscious awareness, but they still influence our judgements.

The ubiquity of unconscious bias was brought home to me recently, when my son texted me a link to a live BBC interview with political scientist Professor Robert Kelly, who was speaking from the office in his home. During the course of the interview the door opens and a little girl in a bright yellow jersey dances in, eager to see what her father is doing. Seconds later, a younger child in a baby walker follows his sister and enters the frame; moments after that a harassed woman of Asian appearance bursts into the office and bundles both children out of the room.

If you'd asked me whether I held racist assumptions about Asian women, I would have vehemently denied it. Yet when my son texted me the Twitter link I'm ashamed to confess that, like millions of other social media users, I too assumed that the woman in the clip was the nanny, rather than the wife of Professor Kelly, a white man. In fact I 'corrected' my son when he referred to the woman as the children's mother and immediately texted back 'Not mum – nanny.' My automatic response was freeze-framed as a text message on my phone; the immediacy of modern technology caught me in the act of unconscious bias.

The cabin crew on Delta DL945 flying from Detroit to Houston in October 2016 made a similar mistake. Following an in-flight call for medical assistance, Dr Tamika Cross, an African-American doctor, offered her services. Initially the flight attendants refused to believe she was a physician. Even when she eventually persuaded them of her professional status, her assistance was declined in favour of that of a white man, who offered no evidence that he was medically qualified. When Dr Cross landed, she posted an account of her experience on Facebook; quickly it went viral, with the hashtag #WhatADoctorLooksLike. The Facebook post elicited a deluge of similar accounts by other women whose claims that they were physicians were initially discounted on the basis of their skin colour, gender, or both.

But it's not just psychologists or airline crew who make these sorts of immediate judgements. Doctors are not immune. Indeed they can't be – because the tendency to reach snap judgements based on stereotypes is hard-wired into all of our brains. The only difference in the medical context is that the people on the receiving end of these automatic responses are typically other doctors and patients. So, for example, Damon Tweedy, an African-American psychiatrist who trained at an elite, overwhelmingly white medical school in the 1990s, was mistaken by a lecturer for a maintenance worker who had come to sort out an electrical problem in the lecture theatre. When Tweedy explained that he knew nothing about the electrics, the lecturer asked 'Then what are you doing here?' All of this took place in front of hundreds of other students, causing Tweedy considerable embarrassment and distress.

And of course, doctors' unconscious biases also get elicited by patients. These biases are about more than race; they may also be about gender, sexuality, age, or stigmatised health conditions such as obesity. In turn, there is compelling evidence that the unconscious biases of clinicians impact not only on the quality of their relationship with patients, and the likelihood that patients will follow their medical advice, but also on the actual treatment decisions that doctors make. For example, a 2012 study published in the *American Journal of Public Health* reported that paediatricians with greater pro-white bias were more likely to agree with prescribing a narcotic medication for postsurgical pain for a white patient, but more likely to disagree with prescribing it for an African-American patient presenting with the same symptoms. Stereotypes about the misuse of pain-killers in the black community got in the way – even though the patients were all young children. The authors of this paper also emphasise how the intense pressure of medical work – clinical uncertainty, a high workload, and fatigue – increases the risk of over-reliance on snap stereotypic judgements.

This is the inescapable reality of medical students' and junior doctors' work. In overstretched hospitals and GP surgeries, as well as in seminar rooms and lecture theatres, they cannot help but see the day-to-day workings of unconscious bias in action.

*

Being on the receiving end of stereotypical perceptions (or fearing that one might be) impairs performance. This effect was brilliantly demonstrated in a set of classic psychological experiments carried out in the Department of Psychology at Stanford University, which used university students as study participants. When the students arrived in the psychology lab, the experimenter (a white man) explained that for the next half hour they would work on a set of verbal problems in a format identical to the SAT (the standardised college entrance test). All of the participants would have previously taken the SAT in order to gain admittance to Stanford.

Each participant was then given a piece of paper outlining the purpose of the study, describing the procedure for answering questions, and stating the fact that test was very difficult, so they should not expect to get many of the questions correct. (Information on the test difficulty was included so that participants' expectations about the test were equalised across the two different test conditions.) In fact, the only difference between the experimental and control conditions were the inclusion of key phrases in the page that described the purpose of the study.

Participants in the experimental group were told that the study was concerned with 'various personal factors involved in performance on problems requiring reading and verbal reasoning abilities'. They were also told that, following the test, they would be provided with feedback which 'may be helpful to you by familiarising you with some of your strengths and weaknesses'. Thus for participants in the experimental group, the test was framed as a test of individual verbal ability.

In contrast, participants in the control group were told that the purpose of the research was to better understand 'the psychological factors involved in solving verbal problems'. Control group participants were also told that they would receive feedback after the test, but it was justified as a means of familiarising them with the kinds of problems that appear on tests, as opposed to giving them an indication of 'personal' strengths and weaknesses, as in the experimental group.

So what happened?

Black participants in the experimental group, where the test was framed as a test of individual ability, performed significantly worse than black participants in the control group – even though participants had been randomly assigned to both groups. The study authors, Steele and Aronson, explained the discrepancy between the two groups in terms of 'stereotype threat', which they defined as 'being at risk of confirming, as a self-characteristic, a negative stereotype about one's social group'. In other words, if people fear that their individual performance might be viewed through the lens of a negative stereotype – their performance is likely to be impaired.

In a subsequent experiment reported in the same paper, Steele and Aronson examined whether increasing the saliency of race (by asking participants to classify themselves according to race, prior to taking the test) amplified anxieties. It was predicted that the impact of stereotype threat would be increased in the 'primed' group, where the issue of race was raised prior to participants taking the test, in contrast to the control group, where participants were asked to record their race after they had completed the test. The results confirmed this hypothesis, as black participants in the 'primed' group performed significantly worse than black participants in the control group.

Stanford University is a world-class institution. In the 2017 Times Higher Education league table it was ranked the top university in the US, and third in the world. Without exception, all of the students who took part in these psychology experiments would have been academic high-flyers. You don't get into Stanford without an exceptional performance at secondary school level – including extremely high SAT scores. Yet tiny manipulations such as emphasising whether the test assesses individual ability, or highlighting cues about race, has an impact on performance. And this even happens to students who have already proven their academic credentials by gaining entrance to an elite university.

Since the publication of Steele and Aronson's study in 1995, there's been a veritable growth industry of research. If you type 'stereotype threat' into the main psychological database (Psychinfo) a list of 923 papers comes up. And whilst the initial study focused on the impact of racial stereotypes on academic performance, subsequent research has investigated many other stereotypes (gender, sexuality, social class, etc.), as well as outcomes beyond academic test results.

Despite the enormous amount of research into stereotype threat, there's been minimal interest in exploring whether it might apply to medical training. Yet given that experiments have shown its impact in so many situations where stereotypes are pervasive – white men compared to Asian men in mathematics; men compared to women on social sensitivity; students from low socioeconomic backgrounds compared to those from wealthier homes on intellectual tasks, etc. – it would be impossible to construct an argument as to why stereotype threat wouldn't occur amongst doctors. And as the initial demonstration of its influence was in a study of academic high-flyers, the notion that doctors are somehow too bright to be influenced by such things simply doesn't hold water.

*

Moving beyond the psychology laboratory, the conversations I have had with doctors over the years often reference, explicitly or implicitly, what it feels like to be on the receiving end of negative stereotypes; feeling that one isn't good enough, or one doesn't quite fit in, or that one has to work harder to prove to other people that one has got what it takes to succeed or that the whole medical training system is desperately unfair. Of course, these conversations haven't only been about race; gender, class and sometimes sexuality are also mentioned. And these different dimensions intersect; consultants would have responded differently to Rahma had she been a man, or from a privileged background.

The notion of 'not belonging' is one that crops up repeatedly. It also runs through much of the wider literature on stereotype threat. And what is one likely to do if one feels that one doesn't belong to the wider professional culture? Stick with one's own. This is certainly what happened to Rahma. She told me how her closest friends at medical school were all young women who came from Pakistani backgrounds, had grown up in her part of London and were living at home. The group had gelled naturally; in the first days at medical school one member of the group had been at secondary school with the cousin of another; there were family and geographic links as well as cultural familiarity. After lectures they tended to be travelling home in the same general direction – so a close-knit group was quickly formed. And the fact that Rahma and her friends didn't feel comfortable socialising in the pub may also have contributed to their relative isolation from the broader medical school year.

Rahma's experience is repeated across the country; students tend to form social networks with others of the same gender and ethnicity. But students don't only learn in lectures – they also learn from their peers. Friends may share hints about new resources, or how best to prepare for an examination. Students within a network also pick up study habits – for good or for worse – from those around them and there is evidence that medical students' choice of friends has a significant influence on their examination grades, even after taking their previous grades into account. Another educational risk, in other words, for marginalised BME students.

I also suspect that the assaults on one's sense of belonging are particularly potent in medicine. If one compares medicine, say, to law – another high-status profession with competitive entry — one finds that medical students spend a huge amount of time in hospital seeing patients (under supervision), whilst law students don't spend a comparable proportion of their time with legal clients. But interactions with patients open up a myriad other ways in which one can come to the conclusion that one has no place in the medical profession. I have never forgotten a brilliant young man from an extremely impoverished white working-class background; his mother was a school cleaner and his father a manual labourer, unable to work because of alcoholism. When he was observed examining patients — particularly if they came from similar backgrounds to his own — he was criticised by his consultants for his accent, or for his less than hyper-formal grammar. The fact that these patients were delighted to be treated by somebody from their neck of the woods didn't alter the negative feedback he received from these senior clinicians.

And it's the same with race. BME doctors will have a different experience of looking after patients than their white peers. One of the incidents that emerged from the inquiry into Cardiff Medical School concerned a patient who refused to be examined by a particular medical student because the student was black. The student was unsupported. More worryingly, some staff felt that this incident should be treated in exactly the same way as if the patient had simply said that they preferred not to have *any* medical student present. Should it really need spelling out, to somebody who trains doctors, that a patient saying they don't want you to examine them because you are black is not the same as a patient saying they don't want you to examine them because you are a medical student?

Then there's the potential for comments from relatives, or from other members of the healthcare team to corrode (or occasionally boost) a fledgling doctor's sense of professional identity. Damon Tweedy, one of the few black medical students in his elite medical school in the 1990s, described his fears that colleagues' views about the black, overweight, diabetic patients they encountered in a rural free clinic would also influence how they saw him – the only black member of the team.

'I had a foot in both worlds – but didn't have two feet in either,' was how he put it.

Of course there is a potential upside. Tweedy also noted the delight when the black people he encountered – patients, relatives, nurses, receptionists, cafeteria workers, cleaners – saw him in his white coat. 'They shared in my achievements and promise like an extended family,' he wrote. But Tweedy went on to stress that, even with the positive feedback, there was a potential sting in the tail: 'Along with the racial pride that came with their praise and adulation, however, I felt an added weight, as if my success or failure would reflect not just on me, but on those who had come before and on those who would follow me.'

*

When we first met, Rahma informed me that she would never be able to work as a doctor. On her first day in her first job, when it became clear to her consultant that she was too depressed to work, she was signed off sick. After a short period of sick leave she returned to work but her self-doubt and depression gradually built up to the point that once again she was unable to work.

The cumulative effect of being viewed through a stereotypic prism probably wasn't the only reason she became so distressed as soon as she started work. Rahma's family background was complicated and, as we saw in an earlier chapter, when a person assumes the role of carer, the residue of how they were themselves cared for in childhood can ripple through their psyche. Faced with the responsibility of looking after sick and needy patients, Rahma's difficult feelings related to her own experiences in childhood may well have been activated.

There's also the issue of wider family responsibilities. Many junior doctors – particularly from BME backgrounds – have described their significant roles in supporting other family members. Understandably, when somebody is sick, if a family member is a medical student or junior doctor, their opinion or advice is likely to be sought. But there is evidence that both the size of the group who are considered 'family' and the weight of the expectations placed on the student/doctor may mean that BME doctors are expected to become more involved in family crises than their white peers. This certainly happened to Rahma; increasingly other family members turned to her for advice and support with their growing list of health problems.

Then there was the issue of living at home. Apart from a short period during her elective, Rahma had never lived away from home. This meant that the quantum leap from medical student to junior doctor coincided with her having to live independently for the first time. 'I'm an adult, why am I feeling like this?' she asked herself. Being surrounded by people who appeared excited about the prospect of starting work made it even harder. 'All I felt was fear,' she told me. Rahma was not alone; other studies have shown that BME medical students in the UK feel less well prepared for the transition to work, although the underlying reasons for this (not having left home before/erosion of confidence in medical school) haven't yet been teased out.

If I look at how Rahma has been transformed, I am clear that her referral to the specialist psychotherapy service for doctors was crucially important. She formed an excellent therapeutic relationship with one of the psychiatrists, who helped her understand why she had been so acutely distressed when she started work. Moreover, Rahma was not alone in finding this specialist psychotherapy service beneficial; a recent follow-up study of 124 doctors found that over 95% who had used the service continued to work and progress in their medical careers, that they took less medication for physical ailments and became more aware of their psychological needs, were less likely to set themselves unachievable targets at work and were better able to access help from colleagues.

I have known Rahma for eight years. Today she is a fully qualified GP; a desperately distressed fledgling doctor has metamorphosed into a quietly confident clinician. Over the past eight years there have been a number of times when Rahma has come to see me. Initially she had hoped to specialise in dermatology; she passed her physician exams, but didn't succeed in getting a training place. After a couple of attempts she changed track and became a GP but she carries a strand of sadness that her first choice of specialty didn't work out. Currently, alongside her clinical work, she has a significant role in research. When she talked about her research interests at our recent meeting, her commitment to this work became clear. Above all else, she wants to ensure that junior clinical researchers, from all backgrounds, are able to realise their potential.

*

'You're wrong,' said the man at the back of the seminar room. 'Completely wrong. It's not the case that white students do better at medical school, or as junior doctors. Not at all. In fact they do worse than their BME peers.'

The speaker, a middle-aged hospital consultant, was one of my students on a Master's course in Medical Education. Despite the fact that I was the module leader, so vehement was his response that I began to doubt what I knew. Maybe I'd got it wrong when I told my seminar group that British students from BME backgrounds got poorer grades than their white peers, and these differences remained, even when you took social class, or the grades of entry into medical school, into account. The issue of race wasn't central to my teaching that afternoon; I'd gone 'off-piste' in discussing the issue in the first place. I backed down.

'I'll check the data,' I told my challenger. So that's what I did.

The following week, I returned to my seminar group. Armed with a lengthy reference list, I felt that I was on solid ground. Although my challenger didn't respond with quite the same level of opposition, I don't think I convinced him that differential attainment actually exists.

To be fair to the consultant in the seminar as well as to the many other white medical students and doctors who remain in blissful ignorance, the problem of differential attainment in the UK is somewhat masked by the high proportion of BME doctors gaining entrance to medical school. According to figures from HESA – the government-funded agency responsible for collecting statistics on the higher education sector – just over one in five (20.6%) of UK-domiciled students come from BME backgrounds. However, when it comes to medical and dental students, the proportion of UK-domiciled BME students is significantly higher: 33.3%. With one in three UK medical and dental students coming from a BME background, it is perhaps easy to see why the myth persists that medical training in the UK has rid itself of racial discrimination. Unfortunately, it is nothing more than that. A myth. Just like the issue of sexism in medicine, the problem isn't access to the first step on the ladder – gaining a place at medical school. It's what happens after that.

So how does the UK compare to the US? The National Center for Education Statistics (NCES) reported that amongst US students enrolled in university in 2014, 13.8% defined themselves as having a 'black/African-American' background. But if you drill down and look specifically at medical school, the proportion of students coming from this group fell to 6.1%. In the US, black/African-American students are less likely to study medicine than other subjects. With Asian students in the US, the situation is reversed. NCES statistics reported that 6.6% of students enrolled in university in 2014 came from Asian backgrounds whilst over three times that number of medical students – 20.5% – were from this group.

A quick glance at the data might suggest that the UK has done better than the US in opening up medical training to BME students. But this would probably be misleading. The UK data groups together students from Asian, African and Afro-Caribbean backgrounds into the 'BME' category. Other studies indicate that young people from Afro-Caribbean backgrounds are less likely to attend university – and are particularly poorly represented in medical school. The fact that a third of medical students in the UK are from BME backgrounds is largely accounted for by the high proportion of students with Asian backgrounds – not by those from Afro-Caribbean homes. Students from that ethnic group – like those from black and African-American backgrounds in the US – are poorly represented.

*

I open my filing cabinet and start pulling out the notes of doctors whom I have recently seen: Sunil, an international medical graduate from India who dreams of being an ophthalmologist, but never gets through the selection process. Then there's Bindu, a UK graduate of Asian origin who is training as a GP, even though her heart had been set on surgery. She knew the competition statistics and in the end decided to play it safe and abandon her surgical ambitions. And there's Tama who is about to be kicked off her training programme in anaesthetics. For each of these doctors, medical work has become toxic. The consultant in the seminar room would probably regard the contents of my filing cabinet as little more than anecdote. But there's a hefty body of evidence to suggest he is wrong.

One of the most comprehensive studies on ethnic differentials was carried out by Kath Woolf and colleagues, and published in the *British Medical Journal* in 2011. Analysing data from nearly 24,000 candidates in the UK, they reached the following conclusion:

Ethnic differences in attainment seem to be a consistent feature of medical education in the UK being present across medical schools, exam types, and undergraduate and post-graduate assessments, and have persisted for at least the past three decades. They cannot be dismissed as atypical or local problems.

In an accompanying editorial to the article, Aneez Esmail, a professor at Manchester Medical School, commented that all medical schools and all specialty royal colleges should analyse their assessment results by ethnic group; they are already required by law to *hold* such data, but Esmail argued that they need to analyse the data and then place the results in the public domain.

How can one disagree with this suggestion? Knowing who gets a particular disease, and in what particular circumstances, forms the bedrock of medical research. One only has to think of the classic research carried out by Sir Richard Doll in the 1950s, in which he followed up 40,000 doctors over a two-and-a-half-year period and demonstrated that as the number of cigarettes smoked increased, so too did the risk of death from lung cancer. Numbers matter not only in medical research – but also in medical education.

In the UK, the GMC is now publishing data that examine the relationship between ethnicity and progression through medical school and beyond. Just as Doll put evidence about the links between smoking and lung cancer in the public domain – thus kick-starting public health campaigns to reduce smoking – the fact that data are publicly available on the GMC website is a vital first step. And the figures demonstrate, beyond all doubt, that there is a real problem.

If one looks, for example, at progression through GP training, 10.3% of international medical graduates (IMGs) are graded as failing to make adequate progress. The comparable figure for UK medical graduates is 3.5%. Similar discrepancies between UK graduates and international medical graduates have been observed in other postgraduate training programmes such as anaesthetics and paediatrics. Being an IMG significantly increases the risk of failure.

The place of primary medical qualification, however, is not the only factor influencing lack of progress; the colour of your skin also counts. This becomes clear when one sees that, on average, British BME colleagues encounter greater difficulties in progression than their white British colleagues. They don't tend to do as badly as doctors who qualified outside the UK – but on average they don't do as well as white doctors. In fact it's almost as if there is a dose effect as in Doll's research on smoking. It's better to be a non-smoker (white) than a smoker (have black or brown skin). But amongst smokers (those with black or brown skin), it's better to be UK born (just puffing away at a few cigarettes a day) than be born in India, or Pakistan, or Africa (having a two-packets-a-day habit). Doctors who fall into that category are at risk.

*

Trying to unpick differential attainment in the American medical system is much harder. One of the key players, the Association of American Medical Colleges (AAMC), puts data in the public domain. From open access data that the AAMC provides it's apparent that black and African-American students tend to enter medical school with lower grades on the MCAT (Medical College Admission Test) than their white peers. It's also clear from AAMC data that black and African-American students who successfully gain a place at medical school tend to come from significantly poorer socioeconomic backgrounds than white students. For example, the largest proportion of black and African-American students come from the poorest backgrounds and the smallest proportion from the wealthiest income group. With white medical students the situation is reversed.

But the AAMC doesn't have responsibility for the United States Medical Licensing Examination (USMLE) that medical students and doctors have to pass, in order to work as a physician in the US. And unlike the AAMC, the USMLE has a very different approach. Information about international medical graduates is shared – and, as in the UK, international medical graduates perform less well on each of the three stages of the USMLE sequence. But the USMLE doesn't readily share information on how US medical students of different ethnicities perform.

Studies of ethnic differences in USMLE examination performance are few and far between. An exception is a 2012 study of students who started medical school between 1993 and 2000, which found that black and African-American students were significantly more likely to fail the first examination (STEP1) than their white peers. Given that students from black and African-American backgrounds enter medical school with lower MCAT scores, and MCAT scores are related to STEP1 scores, this result is not surprising.

The problem is, however, that STEP1 scores then take on a life of their own, as they are used as a screening tool for interviews into residency programmes. As Charles Prober, a physician at Stanford Medical School, explains:

> On one hand we pride ourselves in teaching medical students to use diagnostic tests for their designed purpose, to be critical thinkers and to use evidence-based support to guide their decisions. On the other hand [residency] programs may make career-changing decisions about medical school graduates based on overweighting a screening test in a manner not supported by strong evidence and for which the test was not specifically designed.

Not only is the wrong screening test (i.e. STEP1 scores) used as part of residency selection; it's also a test that is likely to discriminate against African-American applicants: 'When STEP1 scores are used to screen applicants for residency interview, a significantly greater proportion of African-American students will be refused an interview,' concluded one researcher based on applications to his particular medical school.

But we simply don't know how big the problem is across the US as a whole. And the reason we don't know is because of another organisation, the National Resident Matching Program (NRMP). Each year the NRMP publishes a report on the outcomes of the match – a 211-page document in 2016. But the document tells you nothing about race or about gender. Across the whole 211 pages there isn't a single analysis of these basic demographic criteria.

Perplexed, I emailed the Director of Research at the NRMP and asked if the organisation conducted any research into these issues. The same day I received a ten-word response:

'The NRMP does not collect any race or gender data.'

*

We're a little bit ahead of the game in the UK. In 2015 the GMC described their commitment to:

> collecting and publishing a range of outcome data, and analysing it to better understand variation in performance and attainment . . . We're committed to making sure training pathways are fair for all and have a focused work programme to investigate, understand and take action where we find evidence of unfairness or unsupportive environments.

Although the GMC had started researching the causes of racial disparities prior to 2014, undoubtedly the issue gained significant momentum when the British Association of Physicians of

Indian Origin (BAPIO) sought legal redress in the High Court. The matter at stake was whether the final stage of the GP licensing examination should be declared unlawful because it discriminated against BME doctors.

The judge's final verdict was that the examination did not directly or indirectly discriminate against BME doctors. However, following the court case the GMC commissioned two major studies. The first was a comprehensive literature review published in 2015. This review concluded that, although there isn't yet agreement as to the causes of differential attainment, an adequate explanation is likely to involve multiple factors. The authors went on to say that any attempt to mitigate or address differential attainment will have to take account of factors operating at the macro level (policy), the meso level (the institution) and the micro level (individuals and small groups). No simple answers, it seems.

A second study commissioned by the GMC using a focus group and interviews also highlighted the complexity of the issues, but through the use of two words – 'psychologically risky' – the whole debate was radically reconfigured. Differential attainment can't be attributed to deficits in the students, the study concluded; it stems from the fact that whilst medical training is 'psychologically risky' for everyone, the risks are heightened if you don't happen to be white.

The risks that *all* postgraduate doctors face include 'dysfunctional and highly-pressurised environments, bullying, lack of autonomy, lack of work–life balance, and lack of confidence'. That's the day-to-day diet for all junior doctors. But BME doctors – whether from the UK or abroad – encounter 'additional' risks to their progression, including 'difficulties fitting in, unconscious bias in assessments, recruitment and day-to-day working, and occasionally overt prejudice and greater chances of social isolation'. If that list isn't long enough, some special risks faced by international doctors were also highlighted, including 'difficulties forming relationships because of cultural differences and lack of experience of the NHS'.

And the study continued: 'More risks could reduce confidence and motivation,, which could make these doctors less enjoyable to teach, making them receive poorer quality teaching reducing still further their confidence and motivation.'

In other words, accumulated risks produce a potent vicious cycle.

*

Khalid was a surgical trainee who grew up in Saudi Arabia and attended medical school in London as an international student. Tall, traditionally dressed and with a long beard, it was apparent from his appearance that he was a devout Muslim. Although he had an excellent academic record – prizes at medical school, cleared his postgraduate surgical examinations at first attempt and had papers published in prestigious journals – he failed to secure a surgical training position in London, and ended up accepting a place in the west of England. Not only was he separated from his wife and children, who remained in London – he also knew nobody in the town where he ended up working and living.

On the first day the senior surgeon told Khalid that he didn't want him in the operating theatre because his beard was 'unhygienic'. Surgeons with beards can wear beard hoods in just the same way that they can cover head hair with surgical caps. There is no evidence that having hair on one's chin poses any greater threat to patients than having hair on one's head; nobody is suggesting that surgeons need to be bald. Masquerading as infection control this senior surgeon's claim had no basis in scientific fact. Khalid successfully argued his case – but things got off to a terrible start.

On another occasion he was huddled around the computer with a group of colleagues, looking at a patient's X-ray. Apropos of nothing, one of the consultants turned to Khalid and said, 'You people blow people up – you're terrorists.' Nobody said anything, and Khalid felt too frightened to speak out. He didn't want to rock the boat, and find himself labelled as a troublemaker – let alone a supporter of terrorists.

Having been made to feel so unwelcome, Khalid became resentful as well as scared that he would end up with bad reports from this rotation. Desperate to win over his consultants, his solution was to work even harder. But rather than seeing him as a committed surgical trainee, his consultants disliked Khalid's lack of small talk and ostracised him more. Khalid's future in surgery had become risky.

I also struggled when Khalid came to see me. During the first part of the session he talked at me in such a direct and continuous manner that I was left feeling that I couldn't think straight. After about twenty minutes I realised that his manner stemmed from desperation; he was terrified his surgical ambitions could unravel. But just as somebody struggling in the water makes their situation worse by thrashing around, Khalid's frantic attempts to overcome his difficulties were increasing the risk that he would drown.

I had a hunch that the impact he had on me was repeated on a regular basis with his colleagues. So I decided to seize the moment, and talk about it. Choosing my words carefully, I began by acknowledging the racism and emphasised that anybody on the receiving end of such hatred would feel distress. I also told him that whilst I respected his decision not to make a formal complaint, if at any point he changed his mind, I would help find people who could support him through the process. But I went further; I told Khalid that I thought his response (to put his head down and work even harder), whilst understandable, was leading him to be misread by his colleagues. I didn't doubt his commitment to his patients, but I suspected that his colleagues saw him as somebody who only cared about his career. Khalid listened intently to what I was saying and we then discussed ways in which he could better convey to his colleagues that he wanted to be a surgeon because he wanted to treat patients – rather than simply to advance his ambitions.

We only met once. But six months later I received a card in which he informed me he had managed to get a surgical job back in London. Perhaps in that one session I managed to reduce the risk of Khalid's surgical career spiralling rapidly out of control.

*

The racial legacy is not the same on both sides of the Atlantic. As an editorial in the *Journal of the National Medical Association* noted, the history of medicine in the United States has been haunted by a deeply painful past. This includes 'segregated hospitals, limited opportunities for medical training of African-Americans, US government supported clinical trials utilizing African-Americans for human experimentation and reduced access for minority patients to medical care'. In an unprecedented step, the American Medical Association officially apologised to African-American physicians for enabling decades of discriminatory practices against them.

This apology took place in 2008.

In spite of the lack of openness of key organisations what is clear, beyond any doubt, is that African-American, Asian and white medical students in the US don't compete on an even playing field. This was clearly demonstrated in a recent paper in the *Journal of the American Medical Association*. The study looked at racial differences in those accepted into the Alpha Omega Alpha Honor Society. To be asked to join this exclusive club, medical students need to be more than academic high-flyers – they also have to demonstrate 'leadership among their peers, professionalism and a firm sense of ethics'. Why this matters is that being a member of Alpha Omega Alpha is associated with future success in academic medicine. Eleven of the fifteen US Surgeons General have been members, as have more than fifty Nobel laureates. Alpha Omega Alpha are three mighty letters to have on your medical CV.

The design of the study was pleasingly simple – a retrospective analysis of 4,655 residency applications to Yale Medical Center, from students currently attending 123 different medical schools across the US. All of these applications were completed online, and data on the applicants' self-reported race, sex and

age were collected. In addition to this basic demographic information, data on the applicants' STEP1 scores, research productivity, community service and leadership activity were also
extracted. What the researchers were interested in was whether,
after taking all the relevant variables into account, there were
any racial differences in Alpha Omega Alpha membership. And
their results?

> After controlling for numerous demographic and educational
> covariates, we found that the odds of Alpha Omega Alpha
> membership for white students was 6 times greater than those
> for black students and nearly 2 times greater than for Asian
> students.

In an invited commentary to the article the need for tracking
the data on allegedly race-neutral systems of advancement was
stressed.

It's a pity that neither the USMLE nor the NRMP have taken
this message on board.

*

'The first thing that I became aware of in the UK was that I
was a different colour,' Tanisha told me. 'The second thing
was that I spoke differently. Neither of these two observations
had occurred to me before.'

Tanisha was an Indian doctor who attended an Indian
medical school, and then came to the UK as a postgraduate.
Although her secondary school and medical school education
had been in India, the language used in both of these institutions

was English. Tanisha's English-language skills were impeccable, so she was completely unprepared for the ways in which she was made to feel different. 'I became so conscious of my accent that I wouldn't speak in public,' she said. People didn't ask her about the novels she had read (she was a voracious reader) or the films she loved; they heard a slight accent, and assumed that she knew nothing about English culture.

Before Tanisha could work as a doctor in the UK there were also examinations to pass, followed by arranging an unpaid clinical attachment in order to gain exposure to NHS clinical practice. During this period Tanisha had to pay rent, but didn't receive a salary; the money her father had given her ran out and she didn't have enough money to pay for adequate food. By the end of two months, her weight had dropped to 47 kilos.

Each week she spoke to her father in India, reassuring him that she was fine. 'Whether he really knew all along, I will never know,' Tanisha told me.

Four hundred and fifty applications later, she got a six-month job in Wales, in a town where she knew nobody. Without adequate induction into the role, initially she felt completely overwhelmed. To ensure that she didn't make a mistake, Tanisha had no option but to continually ask questions. In turn, her colleagues assumed that she was stupid or ignorant, rather than seeing her as somebody who had trained in a different medical system, and needed a bit of time to find her feet.

And still Tanisha battled on. She stayed late every evening, studied hard, asked for guidance from a fellow international medical graduate, and gradually built up her confidence. Just when she was starting to feel comfortable with the work, she had to move on, as her visa only let her take on short-term contracts. And so it went on for four years, until her visa status changed and she was eligible to apply for specialty training.

Once she started earning a salary she paid back her friends (other international medical graduates) who had lent her money when she had nothing. But she still felt obliged to contribute money to her parents, who were far from wealthy. With all the moving around, she also found herself desperately lonely and isolated. Resisting parental pressure to agree to an arranged marriage, she wanted to fit in with her peers in the UK. Yet in the process, she lost all sense of belonging anywhere: 'I was neither here, nor there,' was how she put it. Exactly the same sentiment as Damon Tweedy made, about his experience as a black medical student in an elite white university.

I have encountered hundreds of doctors from the Indian subcontinent, the Middle East and Africa over the past twenty years. Each one is an individual with their own particular personality, family background, medical training, specialty interests and English-language skills. Some have an easier ride than others once they start working as doctors in the UK. But what unites this disparate group is the fact that the medical profession as a whole systematically underestimates the challenges that these doctors face: inadequate induction; separation from family and friends; being made to feel unwelcome within the medical team; being on the receiving end of barbed comments from colleagues or patients; visa and money worries; concerns about family members that they have left behind – to name but a few of the hurdles they have to overcome.

What makes this collective underestimation all the more shocking is the sheer number involved. Although the number of international medical graduates from Asian backgrounds is decreasing (at least in part, due to visa changes), the contribution that this group makes to the medical workforce is immense. In 2016 the GMC reported that over a quarter of all doctors on the UK medical register gained their primary medical qualification outside UK or Europe. (This is a similar figure to the US, where a quarter of practising physicians are graduates of international medical schools.) When it comes to doctors who are in service roles in hospitals (i.e. those who are working as a doctor without being part of a training scheme), the figures are considerably higher. Imagine for a moment that all these international medical graduates packed their bags and left. Who would care for us?

*

'What happens in medical school is a reflection of wider society,' wrote Professor Aneez Esmail in the *British Medical Journal*. And how could it be otherwise? A medical school isn't a monastery cut off from the outside world. The consultant at the back of my seminar room, Professor *only-interested-in-marriage* and the revue participants at Cardiff University are all giving voice to sentiments that are widely held in society. Probably not sentiments which everybody would espouse – but when we include unconscious bias, from which nobody is exempt, we get a glimpse of the unevenness of the playing field.

As medical school is a reflection of wider society, differential attainment according to race doesn't just apply to doctors; it happens across the whole higher education sector, as well as in primary and secondary school. And it doesn't just happen in the UK or the US; similar gradients have been found in Canada, and Australia and in Western Europe. Across the world, BME students in predominantly white countries face obstacles to their progress.

It's one thing to give a presentation or prepare a report when riddled with self-doubt. That can certainly feel horrid. But it's not the same as having to take responsibility for somebody's life when your confidence has been shattered. This was the situation that Rahma, Khalid and Tanisha, and many other doctors who have come to see me, have found themselves in, day after day. And what's the best buffer against the inevitable stresses of clinical responsibility? Getting support from understanding colleagues. So yet again, BME doctors are disadvantaged, as they are more likely to be isolated and feel that they don't belong in the team.

It's tempting to despair, given the ubiquity of unconscious bias, the depth of structural inequalities and the pervasiveness of differential attainment across the Western world. But there are places where things are done differently. It is possible.

What differentiates these institutions is the scope of their ambitions. As an example (and there are others), over a ten-year period, the University of Texas Medical Branch introduced a raft of significant reforms to change the learning environment, including programmes for students prior to starting medical school; identifying those at risk of struggling with their exams and providing support *before* problems emerged; spending mo hours each week in small group teaching and expanding p support. And the result? The failure rate of African-American students decreased by 93.6%.

More recently, in 2012 a new state-funded medical school in Camden, New Jersey – the Cooper Medical School of Rowan University – matriculated its first class. The mission of the school is to attract students who will serve the local community, 96% of whom are African-American or Hispanic. Like the University of Texas Medical Branch – this new medical school also includes pipeline programmes prior to starting medical school as well as pre-matriculation support. Then there are curricular initiatives such as only having pass-fail grades in the first couple of years, and an emphasis on small-group teaching and peer-tutoring rather than large formal lectures. There's also a mandatory service-learning component from the beginning of the first year so that all students make significant contributions to the Camden community – one of the poorest in the US.

The first cohort at Cooper Medical School graduated in 2012; only one student failed to gain a residency and the school as a whole gained national recognition from the AAMC for its service-learning programme. I strongly suspect that faculty at these institutions don't see an African-American face in the lecture theatre and enquire whether they are there to mend the lights. And I don't imagine that students would put on a theatrical performance that lampooned staff members who were black, or gay, or disabled. I'm not so naïve as to imagine that students don't find themselves on the receiving end of, or overhear, all sorts of examples of unconscious bias. But if there's ough good stuff in the learning environment – supportive faculty and colleagues coupled with plenty of opportunities to develop a strong sense of professional confidence – the risks of failure can be substantially mitigated.

Perhaps, just perhaps, a small imperceptible change is afoot. A 2017 article in the journal *Academic Medicine* has the title 'Breaking the Silence: Time to Talk About Race and Racism.' The article begins with a quote from the African-American novelist James Baldwin:

'Not everything that is faced can be changed, but nothing can be changed until it is faced.'

How true.

8

No Exit

The first thing Bijal told me was that he didn't want to put patients at risk. He ended up double-checking everything he did on the ward because he was so anxious about getting something wrong. The second thing he said was that he was terrified of having another breakdown. These two statements were not unrelated. Bijal was a junior doctor who had a breakdown in his third year of medical school at the point when he started having contact with patients. Although, with extra time, he had managed to finish his undergraduate studies and start his foundation training, the pressure of clinical practice had precipitated recurrent breakdowns. Bijal came to see me four years after he had graduated from medical school; he was working part-time, and still trying to complete his first foundation year. His peers at medical school were way ahead of him on the clinical career ladder, and he had t contact with most of them.

Bijal questioned whether it was feasible for him to complete his first foundation year. The foundation programme regulations state that doctors have to work in more than one placement in order to pass the year, and there was no way round this formal requirement. Yet each time he attempted to move to a different placement he became unwell. However, if you can't get through the first foundation year, your medical career is over.

In our first session Bijal came armed with a shopping list of possible alternative careers, none of which he felt were quite right. Colleagues had suggested medical journalism, or working in the pharmaceutical sector. Or perhaps he could become a dietitian or a speech and language therapist? But he also worried that working alongside doctors in a different healthcare profession might constantly remind him of what he saw as his failure to complete his medical training.

Bijal was stuck.

In our second session, I asked Bijal to draw his 'lifeline' – a visual depiction of the ups and downs of his life to date.

'Every time I change work I get sick,' Bijal told me, looking down at what he had drawn.

But the problem, as he knew, is that you can't progress your medical career by staying put. It was pretty obvious that Bijal had no future in medicine. And towards the end of the session he acknowledged this reality, when he told me that he was '80–90% sure' that he would have to leave clinical practice.

Yet although Bijal was on the cusp of accepting that a medical career wasn't going to work, there was an additional problem. Helping him to move on also involved helping him to cha the mind of his training programme director, who was hell-bent on ensuring that Bijal at least completed the first foundation year. She told me she would feel that she had failed in her duty as programme director if Bijal couldn't take his career this far. But by pushing Bijal to continue, when each change of job ended up with him having another breakdown, the consultant was actually prioritising her own fear of failure over what was best for her trainee.

What Bijal taught me is that leaving medicine is rarely straightforward. Despite the persistent stereotype of the Asian family who put pressure on their children to become doctors, Bijal's family were resigned to him leaving the profession. His parents had seen how unwell he had been at different stages of his training, and they didn't want him to endure a lifetime of mental illness. But even with parental acceptance that a career switch was necessary, Bijal was still unable to decide what to do.

My starting point for helping Bijal was to explore whether there were any aspects of working as a junior doctor that he had enjoyed. For Bijal, all the clinical tasks that he was supposed to be getting on with – taking blood, listening to a patient's heart or chest, interpreting blood test results or prescribing drugs – typically felt overwhelming. But Bijal became quite animated when he described how he liked searching the Internet to find clear information leaflets on relevant clinical topics to give to patients when they were being discharged from hospital. Bijal enjoyed researching good information sources, and helping patients. He just didn't want the pressure of being responsible for their clinical care.

In the next session Bijal told me that he wanted to have predictability in his work as he found uncertainty too daunting. He also wanted the option of working part-time and hoped to find a career with reasonable job security. 'If I do become ill again, I want a job where the work will still be there for me, once I recover,' was how he put it.

I started to wonder whether Bijal would be better suited to working as an academic librarian. Initially the idea came to mind after he told me how much he enjoyed researching information for patients. But I also thought the profession would provide a working environment capable of withstanding periods when he was not well enough to work. Bijal was interested in the suggestion and over the course of the next couple of months went to talk to some librarians, researched different training courses that would enable him to switch profession, and did an internship in an academic medical library.

At a session a couple of months later Bijal reported that he had loved his internship. But *still* he had doubts. What about the length of training? And had we considered *all* the different career options that might suit him? Bijal's intense dislike of uncertainty made the practice of clinical medicine extremely stressful for him. And this dislike also impacted on how he approached a major career decision. He needed to feel absolutely certain that librarianship was the right way forward. Feelings of absolute certainty eluded him.

A few months later, Bijal made a decision. After four years of trying to complete the first foundation year and seeing me quite regularly over a six-month period, Bijal was ready to move on. He emailed me from time to time to tell me abou' his progress. Shortly after starting his new training I saw an advert for a part-time assistant librarian in an academic institution near to where he was studying. I forwarded it to him, and in turn he let me know that he had applied for the post and had been appointed. At the end of the course he contacted me to tell me that he had been awarded a distinction.

Then there was silence for a couple of years, so I was surprised to receive an email from him asking if we could meet up. On the 'no news is good news' principle, I feared that he wanted to see me because this new career had started to unravel. I was wrong. He wanted to talk to me because he was wondering whether or not to embark on a PhD. He also wanted to tell me that while working as the part-time librarian on the evening shift, he regularly found himself going home on the same bus as a graduate student who was using the library. Over the weeks they had started chatting on the bus, then he asked her out, and a few months ago they had got married. As I had sent the job details to him in the first place, he wanted to thank me for helping him meet his wife!

Since leaving medicine he hadn't experienced any periods of serious mental illness. I was delighted to find him in such good health and able to put his intellectual abilities to good use. A few years after that, I bumped into Bijal at a library where I was doing some research. He took out his phone, and proudly showed me a photo of his son.

I needed Bijal's permission before I could tell his story. Recently we had a long catch-up phone call, nearly eight years n from when we first met. I was relieved to hear that he remained in good health, and that he attributed this to being in a less pressurised line of work. He was grateful that he had some balance in his life, and that he was able to spend time with his son. But the topic of leaving medicine was still highly sensitive. 'I hesitate before telling people at work that once I was a doctor,' Bijal said. 'And I don't keep in touch with school friends who went into medicine.'

Exiting medicine can leave lingering feelings of sadness. And this remains true even for doctors whose struggles with clinical responsibility made them seriously unwell.

*

On the face of it, Owen's story was completely different. He was almost at the end of his training when he first came to see me, and his career progression hadn't been complicated by health issues. In fact anyone reading Owen's CV couldn't help but be impressed by his achievements: an Oxbridge graduate with a first-class degree; a PhD quickly completed in the middle of his medical school training; a string of publications in respected journals; postgraduate exams all passed at the first attempt. Without a doubt, Owen was on track to complete his training in psychiatry in a couple of years' time, and secure a consultant post in a prestigious teaching hospital.

Scratch a little bit below the surface, however, and a different picture emerged. In his initial email requesting some sessions, Owen wrote: 'I am finding it increasingly difficult to muster up any enjoyment in my work. My clinical days are mostly characterised by worry before the day starts, followed by sense of relief when it's over (and then more worry about whether I've got everything right).'

I agreed to meet him.

What struck me in the first couple of sessions was the wide disparity between the 'paper' Owen (all the achievements on his CV with a clear focus on completing his training in psychiatry), and how he appeared in person. Face-to-face, Owen was diffident about his accomplishments, and deeply unsure about his future.

Owen had in fact experienced doubts about medicine from the beginning of his undergraduate training. Although at school he was equally strong in science and humanities subjects, his parents (who were the first in their respective families to go to university) encouraged him to opt for science as they reasoned that this would lead to greater job security. Having chosen science subjects at A level, as Owen clearly had the academic ability to study medicine, his parents and teachers all encouraged him to apply to medical school. Nobody seemed to have looked beyond his academic strengths to wonder whether he was interested in, or suited to, the practice of medicine.

Once at university, Owen looked enviously at fellow students in the humanities; they didn't have to put in the same hours as the medical students and when they talked about what they were studying in the college dining hall, he found himself much more interested in their conversations than in those of his medical peers. During the first couple of years at university his motivation nose-dived, and Owen had to resit his end-of-year examinations. It was only in the third year when he faced examinations that would determine his degree class that he started to put consistent energy into his academic work. And when he did, he was able to graduate with a first-class degree.

On the back of his degree results, Owen was offered funding to complete a PhD, which he duly accepted. Again he put his head down, and even though he wasn't particularly interested in the subject, and he encountered terrible difficulties with one of his supervisors, he still managed to get the PhD done and dusted.

At that point, Owen could have abandoned clinical medicine and headed off on an academic pathway. But he felt compelled to continue – a decision which he described as follows: 'One decision at aged sixteen, for people with a certain personality type, and a certain background, can take years to repair . . . Medicine can be very consuming. The hours you work, the constant exams. It's a bit like a cult.'

So Owen continued. After his PhD he returned to medical school to complete the three clinical years; next he progressed through foundation followed by four years as a specialty trainee in psychiatry. In all, he spent a staggering fifteen years pursuing a career that he never really enjoyed. And that's what struck me most forcefully when we met – quite how long he had kept going, despite having doubts from the outset about his career choice.

In Owen's initial email, he mentioned that he was considering leaving medicine. A key issue to review when doctors say that they are thinking of quitting is whether such dissatisfaction is new or long-standing. After the first couple of sessions with Owen, I had no doubt whatsoever that thoughts of leaving medicine weren't a temporary blip on an otherwise committed career pathway.

Some of Owen's doubts related to his chosen specialty – psychiatry. He felt that the specialty was moving sideways, and in contrast to other medical disciplines, there had been few impressive developments over the last thirty years. Sometimes he felt that putting a diagnostic label on a patient's condition and calling it 'personality disorder' or 'major depression' did more harm than good. The patient would have the diagnosis on their medical file for the rest of their life. And he disliked the sense that treating psychotic patients with anti-psychotic medication sometimes made patients feel that the psychiatrist had robbed them of their individual personality. The medication might dampen down the hallucinations or irrational thoughts, but these changes came at a high personal cost for the patient.

'I feel about my work as I do about flying,' he told me. 'There's little inherent enjoyment, and I'm just glad when the plane lands, or the day is over.'

In our second session, Owen talked about how he felt when things went wrong at work. The previous year a patient had died by suicide, and although his clinical management hadn't been called into question, it brought a lot of his doubts about psychiatry to a head.

'It's not the same as a patient dying from cancer,' Owen told me. 'There's just something awful about a patient killing themselves.'

I wondered whether it was the tragedy of this suicide that had led to Owen wanting to change career, but he was adamant that this was not the case. I also wondered whether perhaps he was depressed, and I encouraged him to discuss this possibility with his GP. But what was most striking was how engaged Owen became when he started to talk about the pleasure he derived from writing. I learnt that not only was Owen extraordinarily widely read, but he was also a prolific writer of poetry, short stories and essays. In stark contrast to his academic papers and chapters in medical textbooks, it was the creative side of writing that he loved.

'I'm very aware that I couldn't earn my living as a creative writer,' Owen said. 'There's no money there.'

Just like Bijal, Owen was stuck.

In subsequent sessions, we reviewed all sorts of different options. The most obvious way forward (and the pathway that all his senior consultants were suggesting he should follow) was to become an academic. Owen admitted that he would probably feel less anxious if he traded clinical sessions for research responsibilities as he wouldn't have to worry about the well-being of his patients. But he was fearful that if he went down this route, he might lose the opportunity to leave medicine.

'There's been a pattern in my life of using three-year blocks as delaying tactics,' Owen said. 'First the PhD, then returning to finish my medical degree, and so on. I don't want to make the same mistake now.'

When we looked instead at changing specialty, Owen concluded that he had done so many exams over the past fifteen years that he hadn't the heart to do any more. So that ruled out a specialty shift. Quite by chance, one day I saw a job for a senior editor with a global scientific publisher: I sent the link to Owen, he applied and was duly appointed. But even then, he found it impossible to sever his links with medicine completely. He accepted the new job, but asked the psychiatry training programme to give him the option of returning to clinical medicine in a year's time, should he decide to do so.

Not surprisingly, he didn't return to psychiatry. Two and a half years into his new job he found himself launching a new book series. 'The job demands a mixture of creativity, being meticulous, and seeing where the issues are,' Owen said. He marvelled at how quickly he had been promoted and how natural the different tasks felt, in comparison to the sorts of things he had done as a doctor. In passing, Owen told me that he had recently married.

Working as a doctor had made Bijal unwell, and Owen deeply unhappy. 'I was like a car that was being driven with its hand-brake on,' was how Owen put it. Being miserable at work eats into one's confidence, and corrodes one's self-belief. Conversely, feeling that one is able to put one's talents to good use at work gives one a sense of identity and purpose which can spill over into how one responds to people outside work. I didn't find it at all surprising that the radical changes that both Bijal and Owen made at work were paralleled by significant changes in their personal lives. Both of them found new partners as well as new careers.

*

When I first set eyes on Deepak, my heart sank. Sitting next to him in the reception area was a middle-aged woman who I assumed was his mother. The only other time a medical client had come to see me with Mum in tow, things hadn't worked out well. That doctor was being investigated by the GMC for falsifying research results, and his life had been in meltdown. We only met once, for an initial session. He didn't turn up for the next session, and a few weeks later I got an email from him telling me that he had been admitted as an inpatient to a psychiatric clinic and he would get in contact when he was discharged. He never contacted me again.

All of this rushed through my mind when I first saw Deepak; unthinkingly I equated turning up to a session with one's mother as a bad sign. I feared that yet again I would be faced with a client whose career (and life) difficulties were so profound that there was nothing I could do to help. In the event, Deepak's mother didn't expect to come to the session; she was simply there to keep her son company in the waiting area.

'I feel that there is no way out of my current situation,' Deepak told me in our first meeting. 'I can't go back to my job, but there's nothing for me if I look ahead – no light at the end of the tunnel.'

So what was the problem?

Seemingly out of the blue, Deepak had recently started to suffer from severe panic attacks. There had been no suggestion that he was particularly anxious during the six years of medical school, the two years of foundation training or the earlier part of his training as a surgeon. This was the first time he had experienced any psychological problems.

I learnt in the first session that Deepak's mother was a GP. He had a close relationship with her, and sensibly she had encouraged him to go and discuss his problems with his own GP. Deepak followed this advice and his GP referred him to a psychologist for cognitive behavioural therapy (CBT), prescribed medication, and suggested that he take sick leave for a couple of weeks. It was then that he contacted me and asked for help.

When a client tells me about an uncharacteristic change in their psychological well-being, inevitably I ask myself 'Why now?' So I started to wonder whether currently there was something going on in Deepak's life that might account for these panic attacks. And as is often the case, there were a number of different possible causes, rather than one clear-cut answer. Deepak came from a particularly close family. His uncle had recently died and all of his relatives (and especially his mother) had been devastated. This bereavement happened at a time when he had to change placement in his surgical training, and his new colleagues were unsympathetic. They couldn't understand why the death of his uncle was relevant to how he was feeling. Instead, they constantly criticised aspects of his surgical performance, to the extent that it seriously eroded his confidence. Then Deepak's sleep was affected, which meant that he was going into work feeling exhausted. In turn, this made him feel even less confident that his surgical performance would escape the criticism of his supervising consultants. At this point, the panic attacks started.

I could see how the family bereavement, hostile colleagues, and sleeplessness could all have contributed to his distress. But a deeper answer to the 'Why now?' question only emerged when I stopped asking Deepak about his current circumstances, and instead went right back to the beginning. What had Deepak enjoyed studying at school? When had he decided to apply to medical school? What had drawn him to medicine?

Deepak told me that he came to the UK from India when he was six years old. From primary school onwards, he had excelled at maths and science and this continued throughout secondary school. He couldn't exactly remember when he'd decided to train as a doctor, but for somebody who was ambitious, achieved excellent grades, and also came from a medical family, it seemed like an obvious career choice.

Problems only started when he got to medical school. Throughout secondary school he had striven to be top of the year, but once in medical school he described himself as 'going through the motions'. He wasn't interested in what he was learning, and he did just enough work to scrape through the end-of-year exam. Each year he hoped that what he would learn the following year would capture his interest. But it never did.

Once he started the three clinical years of medical school, things went from bad to worse. Deepak really disliked the way in which medical students can be treated as an impediment on ward rounds and he hated having to 'scrabble around', asking senior clinicians for permission to examine their patients. When I asked him if there was a single specialty that he had studied at medical school that had interested him, Deepak couldn't think of any. Not one.

Like Owen suddenly switching into gear when faced with his final examinations, Deepak crammed like mad to ge‑

through his medical school finals as he was terrified of failure. And he progressed from medical school to being a foundation trainee, in the hope that some aspect of medicine might come along that would inspire him. Plus, he didn't want to let his family down, or feel that he had failed. So with no feelings of excitement about a future career in medicine, he drifted from medical school into being a junior hospital doctor.

In contrast to his feelings about his studies, Deepak had thrown himself into sports at medical school. He had no difficulty motivating himself to turn up for rugby practice and he had captained the medical school first team. Deepak told me about his team's sporting achievements with obvious pride. But his enthusiasm disappeared once he returned to talking about medicine.

Many of Deepak's colleagues on the rugby team decided to pursue a career in orthopaedic surgery. He'd noted that people who enjoyed sports often seemed to choose this option, and as no aspects of clinical work excited him, it seemed as good an idea as any. But entry to surgical training is extremely competitive and Deepak became aware that applicants were more likely to succeed if they had already passed Part A of their surgical postgraduate exams. For the first time in many years, Deepak rediscovered his intense ambition, and he decided that not only would he get Part A, but he would complete Part B as well. This is an extraordinary challenge. In fact the guidelines published by the Royal College of Surgeons strongly advise foundation doctors against attempting both exams as they deem it 'highly unlikely' that a foundation trainee would have the necessary experience to pass.

Deepak not only attempted the challenge, he succeeded. And with this exceptional achievement under his belt, unsurprisingly he got through the surgical selection process. But it was at this point that Deepak's career ran into difficulties; whilst he was delighted by his examination success, he had a growing realisation that he wasn't actually interested in being a surgeon.

Luckily there were things that Deepak did find really interesting. In our second session Deepak told me that in his spare time he read about finance and investments. Recently he had bought a house and was currently involved in its renovation. He loved finding the best contractors to work on the house, and negotiating deals. In fact he'd enjoyed all the commercial aspects of the project, even when it involved researching his legal rights, and getting compensation from a builder whose work turned out to be substandard.

And it wasn't just legal issues linked to the renovation that fired him up. Suddenly he remembered that when he was a foundation trainee he'd challenged the hospital on how they had categorised out-of-hours payments. This was an issue that many other junior doctors had raised in the hospital, but he was the one who managed to get the calculation changed, so that the doctors were paid correctly for their work.

Then there was the issue of a distant cousin who was refused the right to remain in the UK. The matter was referred to an immigration tribunal, but the cousin couldn't afford a lawyer. Deepak researched the case and successfully represented his cousin at the tribunal.

It was law that interested Deepak. Not surgery.

I began to understand the panic attacks.

Deepak was bright, energetic, and hugely ambitious. His family were tremendously proud of his medical achievements. Psychologically he was being pulled simultaneously in opposite directions: part of him wanted to finish what he had set out to do, build on the successes he had already achieved in medicine, and continue in what his family regarded as a 'noble' profession. The other half of him knew that fundamentally he lacked the passion to pursue a surgical career as his heart lay elsewhere.

Given his determination and his loyalty to his family, he had pushed himself for a decade, ignoring the evidence that he wasn't really interested in being a doctor. Someone less driven, less able, and less attached to his family might have given up years earlier. But Deepak would only stop when he became too unwell to continue. I wondered whether the panic attacks were a deep roar from his unconscious telling him that enough was enough.

I met Deepak on only four occasions. By the end of the second session, Deepak started to see the panic attacks in a different light (they soon stopped). Alongside the glaringly obvious need to consider a switch to a legal career, we also discussed a few other options (patent attorney, or working for a medical devices company). By the end of the third session, Deepak had decided to retrain as a solicitor, and by the end of the fourth he had researched a number of different law firms that offered fully funded training contracts, and had already submitted five applications. A couple of months after that, he ·mailed to tell me that he had been taken on by one of the ᵣms, who would completely fund his legal training. He was ᵣg to be a solicitor.

I was delighted but not surprised. Deepak was the sort of person who could push himself to achieve the near-impossible (both parts of the surgical exams) when he wasn't even interested in the subject. Once the passion for the subject was there, as it was with law, he was unstoppable. To use Owen's analogy – Deepak was no longer attempting to move forward with the handbrake on.

I spoke to Deepak recently to ask permission to tell his story. There had been a few hiccups in his training as a solicitor; some of the tasks he was required to do had been quite menial, and not all the partners were committed to training their juniors (much like surgery, in fact). But he'd qualified without any difficulty, changed firm, and now was enjoying working in corporate law. Deepak also told me that initially his family, and in particular his mother, had concerns about his change of career. Why would he want to switch from medicine to law? How could he be sure that he wouldn't want to change again? But they had seen how much happier he was, and now the family fully accepted his decision.

*

It's difficult to leave medicine behind. But as we've seen throughout the book, it can also be difficult to stay. As in my conversation with Deepak, I often have an image of somebody in the middle of a tug-of-war; on the one hand there are powerful forces pulling doctors towards remaining in the profession, whilst on the other hand there are equally powerf forces which pull them in the opposite direction.

The 'remain' forces include fear of failure or of disappointing family members, anxieties that all the years of training will be wasted, pride in being a doctor, uncertainty about whether one will find another job and, if one does, whether one will actually be any happier, an appreciation of the security of medical work, and constant input from senior clinicians saying that it will definitely get better soon. The 'leave' forces include the terror of making a clinical mistake, exhaustion, resentment about the impact of a medical career on one's private life, an unwillingness to move around the country in order to progress one's career, and sometimes a fundamental lack of interest in the profession.

And the end result?

Pulled between equal but opposing forces, doctors stay put.

The rates of doctors leaving medicine – in both the UK and the US – are actually very low indeed. A 2013 survey carried out by a group of epidemiologists at Oxford University concluded that 'UK doctors rarely give up a medical career within 25 years of graduation.' In the US the 2015 Graduation Questionnaire completed by all medical graduates reported that only 0.2% of respondents didn't intend to practise medicine.

That old adage 'Once a teacher, always a teacher' should actually be about doctors, not teachers. Unlike doctors, in the UK nearly one third of teachers who joined the profession in 2010 left within five years. (I should know, as this was precisely how my own teaching career panned out.) But 'Once a doctor, always a doctor' says it as it is. People who start out as doctors tend to end their careers in the profession.

Of course this isn't the message you get from reading the mainstream press. On both sides of the Atlantic, newspapers frequently warn us of a medical exodus: 'Almost half of junior doctors reject NHS career after foundation training' (*Guardian*, 2015); 'Why doctors are sick of their profession'(*Wall Street Journal*, 2014). And in the UK (but not, of course, in the States), the cost to the taxpayer of training doctors who then leave the NHS is invariably mentioned.

It's undeniable that training doctors is extremely expensive. The total NHS investment in each fully qualified hospital consultant is estimated to be over half a million pounds. That's a lot of money to spend on one doctor, if he or she then turns round and leaves the NHS. And with NHS budgets facing unprecedented pressures in the UK, it's not surprising that the issue of doctors leaving the profession makes headlines.

So why do the newspapers consistently get it wrong? One reason, in the UK, is a simple misreading of the foundation data. Each year doctors in the second year of the foundation programme are surveyed about their career plans. It is clear that the proportion of doctors progressing *straight* from foundation into specialty training is in a steep decline (83.1% in 2010, 64.4% in 2013 down to 50.4% in 2016). It is this figure that gets widely reported each year, and contributes to the conclusion that doctors are leaving in droves. It's also clear that the number of doctors taking a break after foundation is on the rise. But the numbers reporting that they have 'permanently left the profession' are vanishing small. In the six years between 2010 and 2016, this fig never reached 1%. (Sadly, the exception to this general rule is the response of doctors from the European Economic Area (EEA) after the Brexit vote. They may not be leaving the profession, but more than 40% of them are considering leaving the UK.)

Other research in the US suggests an additional reason why the numbers of doctors exiting the profession tends to be exaggerated. Using data obtained from the American Medical Association, a group of researchers in California followed up nearly a thousand doctors who had ticked the 'I intend to leave clinical practice' box on a questionnaire. The researchers found that those doctors who were more dissatisfied with their careers were more likely to express an intention to leave the profession. Hardly surprising. But ticking the box didn't predict the *actual* probability of leaving, when the doctors were followed up three years later. 'Self-reported intention to leave practice may be more of a proxy for dissatisfaction than an accurate prediction of actual behaviour,' concluded the researchers.

Yet, whilst it may be relatively rare, some doctors do end up leaving the profession. And when they do, the pain of the decision can linger for years. To quote from a 2004 study carried out by the British Medical Association:

An unexpected finding from this study was how traumatic the decision to leave medicine had been. Many of the doctors interviewed still felt bitter or disappointed and still considered medicine to be their first love. Some were visibly distraught interview . . .

For many the feeling on leaving medicine was of relief, combined with sadness. Sadness because 'it was such a waste' or because medicine remained their real love.

References to 'first love' and 'real love' show the depths of feeling involved. And just like a fraught love affair in which either or both partners half-heartedly threaten to leave on many occasions before making the final break, the whole process can drag on for years. It took Owen over fifteen years before he left the profession. And Bijal, whilst recognising his significantly improved mental health, still expressed sadness at how things had worked out.

*

Zoe was a doctor who came to see me four years after leaving medical school. The university that Zoe attended had an old-style traditional curriculum, with minimal patient exposure early on. Zoe found the first couple of years extremely dull and began to ask herself whether she had chosen the right profession. Like other doctors who have doubts, she took a break between the pre-clinical and clinical years, and by chance got a job as a physician's assistant. This role involved a considerable amount of contact with patients, and Zoe felt she learnt more that year than in the previous three years at medical school.

With renewed enthusiasm for the profession, Zoe returned to medical school in order to complete her degree. She graduated with distinction in both medicine and surgery and wo a number of prizes. The first year as a foundation doctor v extremely tough, but Zoe enjoyed the camaraderie of her colleagues, as well as the sense that at last she was putting what she had learnt at medical school to good use. The thought of leaving the profession didn't cross her mind. The second foundation year was at a different hospital and although she was less well-supported, she was still happy at work. After the foundation programme she climbed up to the next stage of the career ladder, progressing into a two-year 'core medicine programme'. It was towards the end of this phase of her training, at the point when she needed to decide on her final specialty, that she first contacted me.

There were lots of reasons why Zoe had become unhappy at work. She was fed up with working so many nights and weekends, and especially with the impact this was having on her personal life. And whilst she had applied to an oncology specialty training programme, she was unsure whether this was the best way forward. Although she found it rewarding to treat patients with a cancer diagnosis, sometimes she felt that oncologists persisted with treatment when it would have been better to encourage a palliative approach. 'Flogging the patients to death,' was how she put it.

We met once at this stage in Zoe's career, and following the session Zoe emailed to tell me that she had accepted the oncology training post, but deferred starting for a year. She intended to use the year out of training to complete a Master's in medical ethics, and would also work as a locum in order to keep her clinical skills up to date. She needed a bit of breathing space, and time to decide whether or not she really wanted to commit to oncology.

During the first session Zoe had told me that previously she'd struggled with depression and anxiety, and had undergone a period of CBT. We discussed at length whether she might find the psychological demands of treating patients with cancer too demanding. Given her previous history and the fact that she had seemed exhausted by the demands of her core medical training, I wondered whether she might struggle with oncology. Zoe wasn't sure either (hence her desire to take some time out), but on balance she felt that she could manage.

Over a year later when she was two months into her oncology training she contacted me again. This time, it was a very different Zoe I encountered. She was finding the clinical work traumatic; each night when she went home she couldn't stop thinking about her patients. She was also shocked by the physical decay that the disease caused when patients were nearing the end of their life. On reflection, she wondered whether she needed a less demanding line of work.

Building on her recent Master's, Zoe told me that she wanted to find work as a medico-legal adviser helping doctors who were on the receiving end of a patient complaint or who were facing disciplinary action. She no longer thought her job satisfaction was dependent on treating patients and she was interested in the complex legal and ethical problems that medico-legal advisers encountered. Zoe duly applied for a medico-legal job but wasn't appointed. Feedback from the panel was that her heart was still in medicine. Zoe was disappointed, but as she had been told that her chances next time would be greater if she finished her training, with great reluctance she decided to continue with oncology.

The following year Zoe contacted me again. She had been involved in a car accident and sustained significant injuries. After a month in hospital she had moved back home with her parents for a period of rehabilitation. During this time she had done some hard thinking about her career. For the first time in her life, she understood — from the *patient's* perspective — what a huge difference medical care can make, and this had been transformative. In other words, it was being a patient that rekindled her desire to be a doctor.

So Zoe went back to her oncology training. She worked part-time at first, as she was still recovering from the accident, but slowly built up to full-time work. I thought that would be the end of the story. But it wasn't. A year or so later Zoe emailed me again. She was in a particularly unsupportive hospital, and once more was finding it exhausting to witness the suffering that some cancer patients endured. She also didn't see any female consultants whose life she wanted to emulate:

'I don't want to be finishing late, eating kebabs and going home to an empty house,' was how Zoe put it.

So again she was wondering about medico-legal work. Or perhaps she would retrain as a solicitor or even a management consultant. She was desperate to find a career she could enjoy.

'The only reason for me to continue in oncology is that it might open the door to other options in future,' Zoe said.

We discussed at length whether she might be depressed but Zoe felt that this was not the case. So Zoe and I explored her feelings about her current job in great depth, and we also worked out how she could research some of the other options.

At the same time as she was giving serious consideration to leaving medicine, Zoe's training required her to move on to a team in a district general hospital. To her surprise she found the environment much more supportive, and a month or so later, she wrote to tell me that perhaps she had found her niche for the future:

> I really feel that I've looked in all the 'corners and cupboards' now and properly explored my career options, in a way that I haven't before. It was so useful to speak to management consultants, solicitors, etc. and get a feel for what else is out there. I have to say I'm surprised, but very pleased indeed, to conclude that, for me, the grass is not greener elsewhere.

I received that email two years ago. I have spoken to Zoe since, and she told me that she was relieved she didn't end up leaving clinical practice. She's been appointed as a consultant, and combines part-time clinical work with a role in teaching medical ethics. In our recent conversation, Zoe also told me about something that had happened during the year she was studying for her Master's.

One evening shortly before Christmas a twelve-year-old boy was brought into the A & E department where she was working as a locum doctor. He had a fever, felt unwell, and developed a rash. Zoe correctly diagnosed that he was suffering from sepsis and she followed the protocol for the management of this condition in the resuscitation bay. This included applying an oxygen mask, taking blood samples and inserting various lines and catheters into his body. Unfortunately, despite these urgent interventions, the child started to become drowsy, after previously talking quite coherently. Rapidly his condition deteriorated, and the crash team was called. Tragically the resuscitation failed, and the boy died.

Zoe was traumatised by this sequence of events, and her mind kept returning to the fact that in the early part of his treatment he had been able to talk. Different questions kept on circling through her mind: How aware was the boy that he was dying? What happened to his family that Christmas? And, crucially, what else could she have done to save his life?

The death was fully investigated by the hospital, and it was concluded that it could not have been avoided. Zoe was not deemed to have been at fault in any way – but this made little difference to how she felt. She couldn't bear to think about what happened, or to talk about it to anybody. The hospital didn't offer her any support, nor did she seek any for herself. She could now see that it had affected her deeply, both before and after she started her oncology training, and had doubtless contributed to the difficulties she had in her first post and beyond. Six years on she was able to talk about it in a way that previously had been impossible. 'When I'm under pressure, I'm happy to be asked questions about my clinical approach or to ask others for help,' she told me. 'It's made me humbler – a better physician.'

*

Zoe was not alone in experiencing distress following the failed resuscitation of a child. A survey of emergency physicians in the US found that 64% reported feelings of guilt or inadequacy after an unsuccessful paediatric resuscitation. Doctors' hearts are not made of stone.

Of course it is not just doctors working in emergency medicine who suffer when things don't turn out as planned. And unexpected events are far from uncommon in medicine. A recent study of over 600 anaesthetists found that 62% of respondents had been involved in at least one anticipated death or serious injury within the last ten years and 84% had experienced a similar incident at some time in their career. Despite the fact that the majority of anaesthetists had therefore experienced incidents of this type, these events still had the power to cause significant emotional distress: 'More than 70% of respondents experienced guilt, anxiety and reliving the event . . . and 19% of respondents reported never having fully recovered from the event.'

Even when subsequent investigations concluded that the adverse outcome was unpreventable, the majority of anaesthetists in the study still felt personally responsible. What this shows is that the emotional impact of an adverse outcome (feelings of failure, or of being personally responsible) was not linked in a simple way to an independent external assessment of whether the event could have been prevented. Which is exactly what happened to Zoe; being exonerated from blame by the subsequent investigation didn't stop her blaming herself for years.

Twelve per cent of the anaesthetists reported that they considered changing career. A similar figure was found in a study of the impact of perinatal death on obstetricians. What is perhaps most shocking of all is the lack of support for doctors in these situations. 'We have very little in place to allow for proper physician care in the aftermath of adverse events,' concluded the authors of the study of anaesthetists. These words could equally have applied to Zoe.

*

'They have no skin,' Dr H said. 'They are completely lacking a skin.' Then he paused, to allow the seminar audience to reflect on his words.

Dr H was a consultant psychiatrist who specialised in treating medical students and junior doctors and I first heard him speak at a medical education conference. In referring to these 'skin-less' medical patients he was speaking metaphorically – describing those individuals who had to change profession because medical practice caused them excruciating pain. But as soon as he used the term, a roll call of medical students and junior doctors came to mind. I thought about a student who couldn't bear human dissection because she saw the body in the anatomy lab as a person rather than a cadaver. Then I remembered a junior doctor who had to run out of the paediatric ward when confronted with the sight of children experiencing severe pain and another who hated treating elderly patients because all he could think of was that soon they would be dead. Coming face to face with human suffering is difficult without a protective layer – which was the point Dr H was emphasising in his seminar.

But 'skinlessness' doesn't only make it difficult for these individuals to interact with patients; often many other aspects of their life are unbearably painful, including having to consider or discuss a career change. So these medical students and doctors can be extremely difficult to help; they turn up late for sessions, or they cancel at the last minute, often using bizarre excuses. They promise to contact particular people to explore different career options but in the end never get round to doing any of the agreed tasks between sessions. All of this can be extremely frustrating when one is trying to help these doctors move on from medicine.

If somebody was grieving the death of a partner, one wouldn't respond by sending them a link to a dating site. Yet as a practitioner working with these clients it's so easy to fall into the trap of becoming busy and practical – pointing out all the other great careers that they could pursue in future – rather than attending adequately to the distress that the need to leave medicine can cause.

It's difficult to stay with the sense of quite how painful life can be without a skin.

*

Nobody is writing about how distressing it can be when a doctor wants to (or has to) leave the profession; apart from a small-scale study of fourteen doctors published by the BMA over a decade ago, nothing has been written on the subject. And that study, ground-breaking as it was, didn't look at the psychological complexities in any detail.

There's not a single study in a medical journal that describes how doctors can be pulled in two directions simultaneousl· wanting to remove themselves from the burden of clini responsibility yet not wanting to feel disappointed in them-selves, or be a disappointment to their families. And there are no accounts of how it can take years to move on from medicine, or how senior clinicians encourage trainees to continue for just that bit longer, rather than discussing whether it might be better for them to switch career.

A lone voice on this issue is that of the novelist, the late Michael Crichton. In his essay 'Quitting Medicine' he described how in his last year at Harvard Medical School he developed numbness and tingling in his arms and legs which were diagnosed by a neurologist as possibly being a symptom of multiple sclerosis. Following the diagnosis Crichton consulted a psychiatrist, who suggested instead that the symptoms could be hysterical and indicative of underlying psychological distress rather than due to a neurological disorder such as multiple sclerosis. At the time Crichton rejected the psychiatrist's interpretation. A decade later (when he had experienced no further neurological symptoms) he had this to say:

Almost ten years passed before I could look back and wonder whether the decision to leave medicine was so difficult, so traumatic, that I needed the added boost of a serious illness – or at least a possible illness. Because the immediate effect of the terrifying diagnosis was bracing: I was forced to ask myself what I wanted to do with the rest of my life, how I wanted to spend it.

And it was clear to me that if in fact I had only a few years of unencumbered activity, then I wanted to spend those years writing and not doing medicine, or any of the things that colleagues, friends, parents and society in general expected me to do. The illness helped me to stand on my own, to make a difficult transition.

*

Crichton eventually came to understand how difficult quitting medicine can be. But when training senior clinicians I've seen how rational debate tends to fly out the window when the topic of students leaving the profession gets discussed – particularly if the student is academically able. Shortly after working with Bella, the doctor who left ten weeks into her first foundation year, a senior colleague from her medical school contacted me. Would I be willing to see another final year student who didn't feel able to cope with the impending transition to work?

'I'm happy to see this student,' I told my colleague. 'But I've seen so many other unhappy students from your institution that I'd like to come and run a session for senior faculty on early intervention. It doesn't help the students or the NHS if people drop out within weeks of starting their first job.'

My suggestion wasn't well received. Well, not at first. Six months later, however, my colleague got back to me. Could I possibly run a session on how to support those students who didn't think they would cope with medicine, and were thinking of not starting their foundation jobs?

Twelve people came to the training afternoon, all of them senior faculty within the medical school. One of the attendees, a professor of medicine, took great exception to what I was saying.

'It's always better for somebody to finish their medical degree than to change track,' he challenged.

I told the professor about all the people I'd seen from his institution who had taken many extra years to get their degree and then been unable to work as a doctor. He wouldn't shift his views. I was wrong.

Another attendee, also a professor, but not medically qualified, entered the fray.

'I've had an extraordinary career as a research biochemist,' she said. 'But I know that I wouldn't have survived medical training.'

The Professor of Medicine remained unconvinced. At the coffee break halfway through the training session he left.

*

Ironically, it is an ex-nun, rather than a doctor, who has written most persuasively on the topic of changing roles. Helen Rose Fuchs Ebaugh left her life as a Catholic nun in order to become a wife, mother and eventually Professor of Sociology. Using her own experience as a springboard, in her study *Becoming an Ex: The Process of Role Exit*, she interviewed people who had experienced significant role changes in their life. They included women who had been widowed, mothers who had lost custody of their children, people who had changed sex. And doctors who had left the profession. Ebaugh concluded that:

Disengagement from old roles is a complex process that involves shifts in reference groups, friendship networks, relationships with former group members, and most important, shifts in a person's own sense of self-identity.

[Exiters] can feel in mid-air, ungrounded, nowhere. The future is unknown and they no longer belong to the past.

This is an almost poetic description of some of the doctors I have encountered. I have a profound sense of satisfaction that I have helped some doctors to feel less tied to the past, and better able to construct a future. But I am only too aware that there have been others who I was unable to help and whose careers remained suspended in mid-air.

9

Natural Selection

I was once at an event for medical school applicants organised by the *British Medical Journal*. It kicked off with a talk by Ben, a round-faced paediatric surgeon with an endearing smile. If one of my children had ever needed surgery, he was just the sort of doctor I would have wanted them to have; calm, reassuring, kind and obviously highly competent. Almost without exception, Ben held everybody spellbound. He showed them photos taken during operations, and explained that recently he'd saved the life of a seven-year-old boy who had been propelled through a car windscreen at eighty miles an hour. The little boy's insides consisted of 'a puddle of blood', Ben told us, and he put up a slide to prove the point. Four weeks after extensive surgery, the child had left hospital and returned home, with no residual injuries.

About 70% of the audience were young women, nearly all of whom were looking up at Ben with barely concealed adoration. Their male counterparts looked similarly smitten. Everybody wanted to be like him. Everybody wanted to *be* him. He embodied all they hoped to achieve in their working lives. But the more Ben captivated the audience, the gloomier I became. I was the next speaker.

Ben finished his talk to rapturous applause, but as soon as I explained who I was, and what I was going to talk about, the buzz in the room evaporated. That I was the same age as their parents, and a psychologist, made me far less interesting to the audience than Ben. But more than that, it was my central message that they didn't want to hear. If you are attending a seminar on applying to medical school, the last thing in the world you want to sit through is a lecture from a psychologist telling you about all the unhappy doctors she has seen in recent years.

There was muted applause at the end of my talk and I quickly exited stage left. On my way out, a tall middle-aged woman stopped me.

'I wish that had been filmed, so I could show it to the girls at my school.'

She explained that she headed up the sixth form in one of the most academic girls' boarding schools in the country. When pupils were aiming for medicine, they (or their parents) never gave any thought to the issues I had raised. I thanked her, and left – glad that at least one person had found it useful.

A couple of weeks later somebody who had been in the audience emailed me:

Dear Caroline,

I attended the *BMJ* seminar last month where you did a talk on things to consider before applying for medicine.

I am in my last year of school and hoping to study medicine at university. My query is with regard to my health situation. I am currently receiving treatment for anorexia, which I have had since I was 12. Although I am an outpatient, I was wondering whether I would actually be allowed to study medicine. Is there a policy regarding people who have illnesses or disorders that might impact on my application?

I would be incredibly grateful if you could respond to my query. Thanks, Kesia

I thought of the many doctors with eating disorders whom I had encountered, and how in at least some cases promising futures had turned sour. If Kesia was still struggling with anorexia after six years of treatment, would she get through the selection process? On paper at least, the selection panel leaves health considerations to the occupational health team. But anorexia (as opposed to bulimia) is a condition that's hard to hide, so how might her appearance impact on how she was viewed by the panel? Would she be seen as a suitable candidate? If she succeeded at interview, would she pass the occupational health assessment? And if she got through that – how might her career pan out in the longer term? So many questions.

I was unsure how to respond.

*

So who were some of the doctors that Kesia heard me talk about in the *BMJ* seminar?

I started by describing some doctors I've encountered who were nearly, but not quite bright enough to succeed in medicine. Some of these doctors took multiple attempts to get into medical school, and then, once they had been admitted, regularly failed the end-of-year examinations, and had to repeat them during the summer holidays. Typically these doctors had to study much harder than their peers just to keep up, and they had no spare time for social or extracurricular activities. Most medical schools limit how many times a student can fail an examination before they are kicked off the course – but there is also an appeals process which allows students who lose their place on the course to appeal the decision. And that's not all. If the medical school dismisses the appeal there is a national body (the Office of the Independent Adjudicator) that they can take their case to – and often they do.

Students who find themselves in a cycle of repeated examination failure often appeal on the grounds that their performance was affected by depression or anxiety – and this may well be true. But sometimes I wonder whether the depression or anxiety was the cause of the examination failure – or a response to the fact that they knew that despite working as hard as they could, they still couldn't make the grade. I've encountered doctors who have taken over ten years to complete a five-year course. Some of these have qualified in the end – whereas others have spent over a decade failing to get their medical degree.

Sadly, for those students who have struggled in medical school, gaining their degree doesn't mark the end of their difficulties; they then encounter an even bigger hurdle – passing their postgraduate specialty exams. When you're working eleven hours a day as a junior doctor (or sometimes more, as we have seen), it's hard to squeeze in time to study for exams on top of your job. There just aren't enough hours in the day. And if you've only got through your exams in medical school by studying sixteen hours a day, things can fall apart once you start working as a doctor. This was the point I emphasised in my *BMJ* seminar.

Kesia also heard me talk about a different group of medical students – those who struggled with the emotional rather than the academic demands of medical training. Some of these students are academic high-flyers who experienced no difficulty at all gaining a place at medical school. Furthermore, in the more traditional medical school courses where the first couple of years are lecture and lab based with minimal patient contact, these students might also make good progress. But as soon as these students leave the lecture halls and are exposed to suffering and distressed patients – their careers can unravel. In other words, when some vulnerable students start to understand the enormous responsibility inherent in medical work, they can feel overwhelmed. Often these students will then have time out, due to depression and anxiety, or they will have to repeat years because they were too unwell to sit their end-of-year examinations. And this too can drag on for years and years.

Part of the problem is that until very recently, when the GMC started to track doctors from the beginning of medical school onwards, there has been a disconnect between medical school and postgraduate training. The medical schools kept track of their alumni for one year after they left, but they had no systematic way of knowing what happened after that. But I knew – at least for the doctors who came to see me. I always took a detailed educational and career history and before too long I came to see how doctors who struggled to get their postgraduate exams had often had medical school careers that were equally bumpy.

*

Competition for medical school places is fierce. For example, at the University of Oxford in 2015, only 11% of applicants were accepted, notwithstanding the fact that the overwhelming number of these applicants would have achieved excellent secondary school exam grades. Other courses are equally competitive at Oxford; that year applicants to study History of Art had the same chance of being accepted as those applying for Medicine. But there the similarity between the two courses ends. If Oxford gives a place to a History of Art student who turns out to have poor aesthetic judgement, who, beyond the applicant, suffers? But if a medical student struggles to learn the core content of the course, future patients may be placed at risk. 'Selection for Medical School implies selection for the medical profession' is how the Medical School Council puts it. The stakes for medical school selection are high.

In the UK, four-year graduate-entry programmes comprise 10% of admissions. For the remaining 90%, gaining a medical degree takes five or six years, depending upon whether or not a student adds on an intercalated degree. For these students, gaining a medical qualification takes at least five years; often six, if the student adds on an intercalated degree. When you look at the stats, what is striking is the low attrition rate: two studies have recently reported rates of 6% and 5.7% respectively. Similarly, in the US, the Association of American Medical Colleges (AAMC) reported in 2010 that approximately 3% of students failed to complete medical school.

On the face of it, it might seem that the process of selection for medical school in both the UK and US is remarkably successful. The overwhelming majority of students accepted end up graduating. But an alternative explanation is that, from medical school onwards, the medical training system has a profound reluctance, where necessary, to remove those who are not suited to the practice of medicine. This is known in the trade as the 'failure to fail' problem. So what's the evidence for this claim?

In part the evidence is anecdotal, based on the many doctors I have seen over the years who have got through medical school and perhaps even the foundation programme, but didn't have what it takes to progress their medical careers any further. But in addition to this personal experience there is empirical evidence of a significant gap between the numbers of students experiencing difficulties at medical school and the number who end up failing. For example, Janet Yates, a researcher at Nottingham Medical School in the UK, analysed the progress of five consecutive intakes at the school. Yates reported that 12.8% of students at the medical school experienced considerable difficulties: failing a number of examinations, having to repeat a year, serious attitudinal problems noted in their undergraduate records, and suffering from a depressive illness. Just under a third of these struggling students (4% of the total sample) left medical school before graduating. But that leaves 8.8% of the total sample remaining in the system and potentially continuing to struggle, even if they eventually get their medical degree.

There are over 40,000 medical students in the UK. If Janet Yates's figures are taken as representative of medical schools, it means that 5,120 of these students (12.8%) will struggle at some part of their training, with 1,600 (4%) eventually leaving. But it's the gap between these two figures – the 3,520 individuals who struggle in medical school but manage to complete their degree – that I worry about. Doubtless some of them will go on to be good-enough doctors. But some won't.

*

There have been a few studies of doctors who were disciplined for professional misconduct by the GMC (in the UK) or by their State Licensing Board (in the US). Convincing evidence has emerged from these studies that such misconduct was associated with early academic difficulties (in the UK) and prior incidences of unprofessional behaviour in medical school (in the US). So there is good evidence that difficulties in medical school (be they academic failures or examples of unprofessional behaviour) increase the risk of subsequent professional misconduct. However, only a small proportion of doctors – approximately 1% – in the UK and in the US – end up being disciplined by the relevant regulator. Although these findings are important, they therefore don't tell us anything about those doctors who struggle through medical school but whose later clinical performance doesn't warrant a referral to the regulator. Based on my experience of supporting junior doctors who were failing to thrive, I strongly suspect that some of these doctors who struggle at medical school continue to experience great difficulties at work – even if the difficulties are not serious enough to warrant disciplinary action.

From my perspective as a psychologist working within the medical education system, I sometimes witnessed a marked reluctance to curtail a doctor's training. In part, this is admirable; medical training is both long and demanding, and medical students and junior doctors should rightly expect to be adequately supported. But I suspect that other forces are in play as well. Sometimes I encountered a form of institutional denial, characterised by a distinct inability to consider whether the initial decision to offer a student a place at medical school could, perhaps, have been a big mistake.

Jennifer Cleland, an academic at Aberdeen Medical School, is one of the few people who have researched 'failure to fail' within the medical training system. In one study she highlighted how supervising clinicians struggle to give negative assessments to medical students, even when their performance warrants it. One respondent quoted in the study gives a taste of the problem:

> I think part of the difficulty is you know we can all give patients bad news but medical students are potential colleagues and I think we're very bad at communicating that sort of thing to our colleagues.

I find this extraordinary; what this doctor is saying is that she finds it easier to tell a patient that they are dying than to tell a medical student that they are failing. It's another example of the way doctors unconsciously separate themselves from their patients – seeing them as belonging to a different group – in order to manage the inevitable anxieties of clinical work. And the result of this unconscious manoeuvre is that delivering catastrophic news to a patient becomes easier than talking to a medical student about their serious career difficulties. Other issues that supervising clinicians mentioned in Cleland's study included lack of time, and lack of clear guidance on standards. Senior clinicians can feel unsure whether the clinical performance they observe when a student is with them constitutes a failing grade or not. This is hardly reassuring for future patients who might be treated by these medical students once they qualify.

In a later review spanning studies in the UK as well as North America, Cleland goes a step further, and questions the whole approach to remediating underperforming medical students:

> The ethics of supporting students to progress to the next stage of training only to continue to perform poorly are, at best, questionable. It is also debatable whether scarce faculty resources should be used to support progression without improvement, which may take weak students further towards registration as potentially weak doctors when the evidence suggests that faculty members find it harder to fail senior students.

This is a step in the right direction – but it still doesn't go far enough. What never gets said is that it is *inevitable* tha some medical students will fail. Acknowledging this truth appears to be a step too far for the medical training system. Yet in order for *all* medical students to be perfectly suited to their chosen course, two conditions would have to hold true. First, the process of selection into medical school would have to be 100% accurate; and secondly, students would never change throughout the four, five or six years of their course. Clearly both assumptions are absurd, and even if the numbers are not huge, there are invariably going to be some individuals in the system – at medical school, and beyond – who shouldn't be there.

This 'failure to fail' doesn't occur only in medical training; it has been noted throughout the health and caring professions. Undoubtedly in both the UK and the US, a growing fear of litigation complicates the picture. Failing students can seek legal redress from the medical school, and gaining a reputation for removing students from the course doesn't sit well with the financial need medical schools have to attract future applicants. But the unwillingness to tackle the issue of medical students who are unsuited to the practice of medicine doesn't only pose risks to future patients – it also creates misery for the students themselves. Some of the students and doctors I've encountered should never have been allowed to remain in the system for so long. I wouldn't want Kesia to suffer such a fate.

*

Wherever in the world one is applying to train as a doctor, significant weight will be given to one's academic achievements.

How that achievement is measured, the final weight that is attached to it in the overall selection decision, and what other factors are also taken into account, differ considerably between different countries and even between different universities within the same country. But everywhere in the world, prior academic achievement will form a central piece of the jigsaw that medical school selectors piece together when making their decisions.

In the US all prospective medical students have to sit MCAT (the Medical College Admission Test), a standardised computerised assessment. In medical schools across the country, admissions panels attach great weight to MCAT scores, and they have routinely been shown to predict results on the first set of national examinations (STEP1) that medical students take at the end of their second year. But all this means is that results on one computerised standardised assessment (MCAT) are significantly correlated with results on another computerised standardised assessment (STEP1) taken two years down the line. In contrast, the ability of MCAT scores to predict later clinical performance as a doctor seems, at best, to be extremely weak. (The examination was revamped in 2015, and now includes sections on psychology and sociology. It's too early to know whether these new sections will better predict future clinical performance as a practising doctor.)

In the UK, A-level grades are used to assess academic potential for medical school. A-level grades predict both written and practical tests that are taken later during medical school. Chris McManus, a professor of medical education at University College London, uses the metaphor of the 'academic backbone' to describe the idea that, in medical education, current learning and achievement is critically dependent upon achievement at earlier stages. For McManus, this 'backbone' comprises 'the accumulation of "medical capital", that set of knowledge, theories, experience, understanding and skills that comprise successful medical practice'.

According to this argument, it is essential that adequate weight is given to the academic achievement of applicants to medical school; if your backbone is weakened, you are not going to be able to stand up, let alone run. McManus also counters the frequently levelled criticism that choosing medical school applicants on the basis of school exam grades leads to the selection of students who are good at passing exams, but not necessarily good at the practice of medicine. He points out that 'knowledge is generally preferable to ignorance, and clinical knowledge underpins clinical practice'. As a patient, it would be difficult to disagree with this; who wants to be treated by an ignorant doctor? And when I encounter doctors who have struggled academically from the beginning of their medical training, McManus's warning that one needs to give adequate attention to prior academic achievement rings true.

But of course, academic achievement isn't the whole story. Whilst as patients we want knowledgeable doctors rather than ignorant ones, we also need our doctors to have a whole host of other qualities such as empathy, an ability to handle pressure, to work well with their colleagues, and personal integrity. Academic achievement alone isn't enough, when it comes to selecting doctors.

Basing selection decisions on academic achievements also introduces a social bias into the process because applicants from higher-income families tend to achieve better A-level grades. For example, a national survey of first year foundation doctors found that 31% attended a private school whilst only 7% of children in the UK were educated in the private sector – more than a fourfold over-representation. A similar social bias is seen in the US: the percentage of medical students from the highest 20% of parental incomes has never been lower that 48%, whilst the percentage of medical students from the lowest 20% of parental incomes has never exceeded 5.5%.

Part of the problem, however, is that as medical schools have traditionally demanded the highest academic standards, there are little data available on whether it is feasible for a medical school to lower its academic entrance grades and still produce competent doctors. King's College London, however, since 2001 has admitted students from low-achieving secondary schools, with lower grades than those normally required for medical school admission. Students admitted to this Extended Medical Degree Programme (EMDP) have an extra year to gain their final medical qualification.

Perhaps not surprisingly, given the association between A-level grades and medical school exam performance, EMDP students are significantly more likely to fail finals. McManus therefore cautions against lowering entry grades without research into how much they should be reduced, and for which groups. A depressing conclusion – and also, perhaps, an incomplete one. Because even though EMDP students are more likely to fail finals than their peers who were admitted with higher A-level grades to the standard five-year programme, there is some suggestion that they are also over-represented in the most highly performing students. If you lower the entry grades for students who went to poorly performing schools you will increase the proportion of failures, and you will also identify brilliant students who otherwise would never have been given the chance to train as doctors. Tough choice. Isn't there a better way of selecting the future medical workforce?

*

The holy grail of medical selection is a test that measures the potential of an applicant *independent of* the educational opportunities that the applicant has previously experienced. In this way, so the argument goes, able applicants can be identified whose secondary school grades were reduced because of the poor quality of education that they received. In the UK, two such tests have been devised – the UKCAT (United Kingdom Clinical Aptitude Test) and the BMAT (BioMedical Admissions Test). But do these tests provide an objective measure of 'potential', as the test suppliers claim? Do they tell us any more about the candidate than their A-level grades? And does their use lead to the selection of a more socially diverse set of medical students?

A five-year study of over six thousand entrants to medical school in the UK provides some good answers. What the study found was that UKCAT scores were significantly predictive of later performance at medical school, even when prior A-level results were taken into account. In other words, UKCAT results *did* add value to the selection process. The authors also argued that relying on UKCAT scores rather than A-level results could help to widen participation, as the former seems to be less influenced by the quality of secondary school education. So good news on both counts.

The evidence about BMAT is much less impressive. The only part of the BMAT test that predicts later performance at medical school is the knowledge component. This part of the test is close in structure to a standard academic test such as A levels, and students who do well on it also do well in their A levels. So as yet there's no evidence that the BMAT provides an education-free test of 'potential' as the test suppliers claim, or will do anything to widen participation. Is it a coincidence that this is the entrance test favoured by elite medical schools in the UK such as Oxford, Cambridge and Imperial College?

Over the years I have spent supporting doctors, I've certainly encountered some exceptionally able doctors from working-class backgrounds; doctors whose parents were van drivers, or shop assistants, or who worked in a factory. But they are very much the exception rather than the rule. And as we have seen in earlier chapters, doctors who don't come from professional backgrounds often struggle to feel that they fit in. On ward rounds consultants might criticise their accent or grammar and they often tell me that they feel less confident than their privately educated colleagues.

But it's not just my own impression that medicine in the UK remains elitist; in 2012 the profession was named and shamed because of its poor record on social mobility. The Independent Review on Social Mobility and Child Poverty had this to say:

> Medicine lags behind other professions . . . It has a long way to go when it comes to making access fairer, diversifying its workforce and raising social mobility . . . The profession itself recognises that the skills which modern doctors require include far greater understanding of the social and economic background of the people they serve . . . It now needs to be matched by action. Overall, medicine has made far too little progress and shown far too little interest in the issue of fair access. It needs a step change in approach.

In terms of widening access, the profession isn't keeping up. And this really matters, for a number of reasons. First there is the issue of social justice, and the desirability of having a fairer, more fluid society. According to this argument, the cohesiveness of society is at stake if individuals from particular groups feel that they have no chance of improving their social circumstances, even if they have the ability to do so. Then there is evidence that diversifying the medical workforce (be it in terms of social class or ethnicity) produces doctors who are more likely to work in the communities from which they were drawn. So for example a Scottish study found that GPs from less affluent backgrounds were more likely to work in GP practices serving the most deprived communities, compared to colleagues who came from more middle-class families. And it also seems that students who study in a more diverse medical school end up having more positive attitudes towards patients from minority groups than those who study in more ethnically homogeneous medical schools.

*

In response to the damning criticism, the Medical Schools Council launched an initiative to make selection into the profession fairer and more transparent. Previously medical schools had been criticised for the somewhat opaque way in which selection panels operated. Beyond academic excellence, what else were they looking for in an applicant? In order to counter the charge of lack of transparency, in 2014 the Medical Schools Council compiled a list of the key skills and attributes needed to study medicine.

The list kicks off with 'motivation to study medicine and genuine interest in the medical profession', which is a reasonable starting point. Next is 'insight into your own strengths and weaknesses', which also seems sensible. In total, seventeen personal qualities are listed. Perhaps I'm reading more into the order than is warranted, but I can't help feeling an element of disquiet that 'empathy' and 'honesty' are at the bottom of the list. Studies that have asked patients what they look for in their doctor indicate markedly different priorities, with empathy coming near the top of the list.

Whilst I might quibble with the order, overall the list of attributes contains those that people hope to see in their doctors. But the key question is: how can they best be evaluated in a medical school applicant? Traditionally in the UK and in North America, medical schools have used a combination of written personal statements submitted in advance by the applicant, and interviews. But what's the evidence that these methods work?

A major review of best practice in the selection of medical students commissioned by the GMC had this to say:

> Research evidence suggests that autobiographical submissions (like personal statements) are more susceptible to contamination and input from third parties than many other common selection methods, which disadvantages applicants from lower socioeconomic groups who are less likely to have the appropriate networks and resources to provide this.

The GMC report concluded that evidence supporting the utility of personal statements was 'limited'. Nowadays, the Medical Schools Council produces a guide that lists the selection methods used by every institution in the UK. The 2017 Guide shows that the majority of UK medical schools no longer score personal statements – so clearly they have taken recent research findings on board. But what about being interviewed by a panel? Is this method any better at predicting who will turn out to be good doctors?

*

My experience of sitting on an interview panel at a London medical school was not encouraging. I was shocked when another panel member marked an applicant down because she had only decided to apply to medical school in the last nine months. Implicitly this panel member was equating

duration of the desire to apply for medicine with the robust-
ness of that decision. This assumption runs counter to the
results of a study that asked over two thousand eleven-
year-olds about their career plans and mapped their
responses to standardised tests of ability. The study found
that 10% of the sample of eleven-year-olds expressed an
interest in medicine, but this interest was not associated
with high educational attainment or cognitive ability.
Children in this sample seemed not to be making very
robust career decisions (and why should they? Eleven years
old is definitely too young to be making such a choice).
But my colleague wanted to mark down an applicant
because she had made her career choice as a seventeen-
year-old, rather than as a younger child.

Then there's the whole issue of unconscious bias. There's
been little research that has looked specifically at the impact
of unconscious bias in medical school admissions, but as it's
known to be a significant factor in interviews for other
professions, there's no reason why doctors would be exempt.
Some medical schools such as the Icahn School of Medicine
in New York are doing unconscious bias training for all
interview panel members – and there is good evidence that
this can make a difference. For example, in a recent study
in a state medical school in the Midwest all 140 members of
the admissions committee were taught about unconscious
bias and took the implicit association test – an assessment
of unconscious racial bias. All members were found to have
significant levels of unconscious preferences for white
people. Following this training nearly half of the committee

members reported that they were conscious of their biases during the next admissions cycle and the class admitted that year was the most racially diverse in the history of the medical school.

I also found from my experience as a panel member that traditional medical school interviews don't explore a candidate's motivation in any real depth – despite the fact that this is the personal quality that tops the list of the Medical Schools Council. This was definitely what had happened with Kevin, the doctor whose sister died of leukaemia.

Medicine wasn't actually Kevin's first choice of career; he started off training to be an engineer and only considered switching to medicine after his sister became ill. Visiting her in hospital during her treatment, the idea of training as a doctor took hold. Sadly the treatment didn't work for Kevin's sister and a couple of years after diagnosis, she died. Immediately after her death, Kevin applied to medical school, even though the doctors treating his sister strongly advised him to wait a couple of years.

So for Kevin, like some other doctors we've met in earlier chapters, the initial motivation to study medicine was intimately linked to illness within the family. But the interview panel didn't dwell on this link, which is in stark contrast to what happens when you apply to train as a psychologist or psychotherapist. In interviews for those professions, one's own motivation for choosing that particular career will be put under the microscope. Personal or family experience of mental illness won't rule one ut of the profession but there is an explicit expectation that applicant should understand the links between things that have happened to them in the past, and their desire to help people experiencing mental health problems.

In medical school interviews it's not considered vital that an applicant has fully explored the way in which personal and family experience of illness might be related to their decision to train as a doctor. But such an understanding is essential because when people are faced with a tragedy, the desire to make sense of the experience, or to extract something constructive out of it, can be overwhelming. Somebody you love dies of cancer – you run a marathon to raise money for cancer research, or for the hospice that cared for your loved one at the end of their life. A cyclist gets crushed by a lorry – you campaign for separate cycling lanes, or heftier penalties for careless lorry drivers. You've just graduated with a good degree in engineering and your sister dies from leukaemia so you decide to capitalise on your scientific potential and train as a doctor.

'By choosing medicine, something good could come out of my sister's death' was how Kevin explained it to me.

Making a career choice like this isn't necessarily problematic. However, it *can* be, as it was with Kevin. Because in Kevin's case the human desire for something constructive to emerge from a personal tragedy overshadowed an appreciation of the ways in which he might struggle with medical work. Undoubtedly he had the academic potential – he had top A-level grades and a first-class degree in engineering. But Kevin told me that he found it extremely upsetting to witness human suffering and he struggled with the responsibility inherent in medical work. Even before Kevin started medic school he had doubts about whether he was psychologically suited to the profession; doubts which were not fully explored at the interview.

*

Panel interviews for medical school places are on the way out, anyway. In their place, applicants are assessed by 'multiple sample' methods that have been used for many years to assess the clinical competence of medical students later on in their training. So for example when a student's ability to communicate effectively with a patient is assessed in medical school, they will be observed rotating through a large number of 'stations', each one consisting of a different communicative task. In one they might have to break bad news to an actor-patient whilst in another, they might have to placate an actor role-playing an angry relative.

The reason that students are observed carrying out multiple tasks is that an individual's performance is influenced far more by the specifics of the task than one intuitively expects; a candidate can do brilliantly in one station but far less well in another, even though one might have predicted that both tasks draw on a similar underlying skill. But it was not until 2004 that Professor Kevin Eva and his colleagues at McMaster University in Canada adapted these methods, which have become a ubiquitous feature of medical school education, for use in the *initial* selection of medical students.

What Eva ended up with was ten different stations, assessing ferent skills — the so-called multiple mini interview (MMI) format. Each station lasted eight minutes, followed by a two-minute interval during which interviewers completed standardised evaluation forms, and candidates read the details of the next station. Assessors stayed put, while candidates rotated between the stations. With this MMI format candidates are therefore observed for eighty minutes (ten stations each of eight minutes). As a comparison, with traditional panel interviews, each candidate was typically given no more than twenty minutes – so the MMI format quadruples the time spent with each candidate.

In two of the ten stations, candidates were asked typical interview questions: 'Why do you want to be a physician?' and 'What experiences have you had (and what insights have you gained from these experiences) that led you to believe you would be a good physician?' But the other stations were very different. A candidate's capacity for ethical decision making was assessed by giving them the following scenario:

Dr Cheung recommends homeopathic medicines to his patients. There is no scientific evidence or widely accepted theory to suggest that homeopathic medicines work and the doctor doesn't believe them to. He recommends homeopathic medicine to people with mild and non-specific symptoms such as fatigue, headaches and muscle aches, because he believes it will do no harm, but will give them reassurance.

The candidate is instructed to consider the ethical problems that Dr Cheung's behaviour might pose and discuss these issues with the interviewer. (I find it surprising that an obvious

Chinese name was chosen. But perhaps this was done deliberately in order to see if candidates trotted out any racist stereotypes. Or, alternatively, to see whether an outstanding candidate was able to make subtle observations about the expectations that patients from different cultural backgrounds might bring to the clinical encounter.) The second station on ethical decision making asked the candidate to consider whether physicians should provide circumcisions for religious as opposed to medical reasons.

In the two communication skills stations, actors were used. In one, the candidate was told:

Your company needs both you and a co-worker (Sara, a colleague from another branch of the company) to attend a critical business meeting in San Diego. You have just arrived to drive Sara to the airport. Sara is in the room.

What the candidate wasn't told is that Sara (played by an actor) is somebody who has developed a fear of flying, following the September 11 attacks. In this particular station, the interviewer doesn't ask any questions, but instead observes how empathic the candidate is, and how well they manage to communicate with their fictional 'colleague'. The other communication skills station involved the candidate explaining to Tim (also played by an actor) that they had crashed into his BMW in an underground car park.

A candidate's critical thinking was assessed in one station ⸍ providing them with a short piece of information about ῀ficial sweeteners, taken from the Internet, which they then had to critique. Another station assessed knowledge of the healthcare system; so, for example, they were asked their views on whether patients should be charged a small fee each time they went to visit the doctor, to discourage unnecessary visits.

The day-to-day stuff of medical work certainly requires doctors to have a firm grounding in medical science but they also need to communicate well with their patients, and with the patients' relatives, who can be distraught, or furious, or in despair. They need to work well with their colleagues who may be stressed and burnt-out, and make tough choices between competing priorities. They need to understand the implications and the inevitable constraints of the particular healthcare system in which they practise. And the MMIs try to assess whether the applicant might be able to carry out these sorts of task in future.

*

Thirteen years after they were introduced in Canada, MMIs have become standard practice throughout the world. In the UK, they were piloted by Dundee Medical School in 2008, and formally adopted in 2009. Ready-made MMIs don't exist. Each time they have been incorporated into the admissions process the content of each station has to be worked out, matched to the precise priorities of each medical school. There's often political work that needs to be done to bring the sometimes crusty members of the medical school's admissions committee on board. Assessors and any actors need to be recruited and trained. And space needs to be found.

As an assessor on an MMI at a London medical school I have seen how the whole enterprise has to be coordinated like a military manoeuvre; it's a huge amount of work. The questions have to change each year, so that the scenarios don't leak out and coaching companies don't get rich training candidates in model answers. But having sat on old-style interview panels and also MMIs, it's clear to me that the latter assess a broader range of skills, and also allow each applicant to be observed for a longer period of time.

Thirteen years after they were first introduced, sufficient evidence has accrued to demonstrate that MMIs improve the selection process. As an example (and there are many others from around the world), when Kevin Eva followed up the original cohort, the MMI scores were found to be the best predictor of scores on clinical performance assessments, clerkship ratings by their supervisors, and clinical aspects of the Canadian Medical Licensing exam.

In 2011, the great and the good in the world of medical education got together and produced a consensus statement and recommendations on medical student selection. Globally they concluded that: 'There is evidence of the predictive validity of the multiple mini-interview . . . Furthermore there is evidence on this issue from outside of North America. There is not much evidence of the credibility of interviews, personal statements and letters of reference.'

Dundee was the first medical school in the UK to get the message, and thirty-one others have now followed. Only six medical schools in the UK are still using panel interviews ¬ the 2017 recruitment round. Four of these institutions

(Oxford, Cambridge, Imperial and University College London) also use the BMAT to assess 'aptitude'. Except, as we now know, it assesses scientific knowledge – a metric that is inevitably influenced (like panel interviews) by the sort of school that the applicant had the luck, or misfortune, to attend.

'Around the world, medical schools' desire to apply the similarly rigorous standards of evidence to their admissions processes that they have typically applied to their clinical practice, have resulted in the typical interview being replaced by MMI,' wrote an optimistic proponent of MMIs. Not everywhere, it would seem. Not only are there a small number of medical schools in the UK (and elsewhere) that are ignoring the compelling evidence that old-style methods don't work. Some of these institutions are the very same ones that are carrying out research showing the flaws in the old methods – yet the medical school admissions panels don't seem to take any notice of their colleagues' published findings. As an example, Chris McManus at UCL has contributed to the global consensus statement on best practice in selection, but his medical school still uses panel interviews. He has highlighted the limitations of BMAT, but that's what the admissions committee at UCL medical school has chosen to use.

In a similar vein, Donald Barr, a paediatrician writing in *The Lancet* described how research from the psychology department at University of California, San Francisco, showed that MCAT and undergraduate science scores failed to predict later clinical performance at medical school. But he sat the admissions committee at UCSF Medical School without ever being informed of this research.

*

A colleague once told me about a medical student who had been granted a place, despite failing to get the required grades, because his mother had unexpectedly died during the period when he was sitting his A-level exams. Fair enough, you might think. Except that it later transpired that his mother hadn't died; the story was a lie. Yet he was still allowed to continue at medical school. A couple of years into the course when the student was failing badly he was summoned to a meeting with the Head of Year. On the day of the meeting he told his Head of Year that he couldn't come because he had an urgent appointment with another faculty member. It later transpired that this was also a lie. But still he didn't lose his place.

This was a number of years ago and my sense is that nowadays medical schools are more stringent about managing students who are dishonest. Unprofessional behaviour (such as lying) as a student has been shown to increase the risk of subsequent disciplinary action by the medical regulator once the student has qualified. Thus overlooking this sort of dishonesty is short-sighted in the extreme – particularly because you can't get much of a handle on this personal quality by direct questioning at an interview. What is a dishonest person likely to do, if questioned about their honesty? Lie. So simply asking won't work. And in an MMI format, the stakes are so high that, even if an applicant often resorts to lying in real life, they will probably tell the truth in that context. Instead, seemingly minor examples of dishonesty throughout the course need to be treated extremely seriously.

But from my perspective, the Achilles heel of medical school selection is its inability to assess emotional resilience. Of the many struggling doctors I have encountered over the last decade, a small proportion probably didn't have the cognitive ability to succeed in medicine, and a slightly larger proportion came to the conclusion that they weren't sufficiently interested in medical science to continue in the profession. The remainder found medicine too emotionally demanding. Often (as we have seen in earlier chapters) their difficulties were due to temporary factors: personal illness, family bereavement, relationship breakdown, being placed in a particularly hostile work environment, lack of support from colleagues or being asked to carry out tasks for which they were inadequately trained. Sometimes the distress was due to them being in the wrong branch of medicine. But for at least some of these doctors medicine, in any shape or form, was too much for them to manage.

Should the medical school selection process have weeded them out?

All applicants to medical school have an occupational health assessment. In most cases health conditions will not bar somebody from becoming a doctor, because 'reasonable adjustments' to their training can be made. Health matters are also considered separately from the selection process. According to the guidance published by the GMC and the Medical Schools Council, a history of serious health issues, including mental health conditions, will not jeopardise a career in medicine unless the condition impinges on professional fitness to practise:

> Medical schools should explain that mental health conditions are common in medical students and that support is available. In almost every case, a mental health condition does not prevent a student from completing his or her course and continuing a career in medicine.

I've encountered many doctors who had already experienced episodes of mental illness prior to entering medical school, and occupational health allowed them to pursue medical training. Often this has worked well, but sometimes it hasn't. And occupational health can't be expected to screen out all those students who won't cope with medicine *before* they start their course; some doctors only develop a mental illness a couple of years into medical training, so there would not have been any prior illness to declare when they first applied to medical school.

What about the interview process? Is that a way of identifying those applicants who might not cope with medical training?

There are exceptional cases where the answer is 'yes'. For example, as part of an MMI I once assessed an applicant who shook so much with terror that she couldn't utter a word. I don't think I'm intimidating, and I didn't have a similar effect on any other applicant; I took great pains to make all applicants feel as comfortable as possible. When it became apparent that she was unable to speak I gently told her to take her time, and that I would wait for an answer until she was ready.

But she never got to the point where she was able to answer the question.

This case was highly unusual and is a rare example of when the MMI method demonstrates that somebody may struggle to cope with medicine. It would be difficult to devise an effective MMI task that directly assessed emotional resilience (although a few medical schools have tried). Other medical schools have advocated using a screening questionnaire. However, I suspect that applicants who are desperate to gain a place will answer these questions by thinking about what the assessment panel is looking for, rather than giving answers that actually reflect how they typically respond in stressful situations.

It's not that emotional resilience cannot be measured. Organisations that assess whether staff will cope with extremely demanding assignments (working in the field during the Ebola crisis, for example) have developed sophisticated questionnaires. The breadth of issues these cover is astonishing: childhood traumas; past and current relationships with family; current support from friends; relationship with one's partner (or lack of relationship); previous episodes of depression; sleep difficulties; current and past ability to look after oneself appropriately, etc.

If medical schools' admission panels asked these sorts of questions, I suspect they would be able to identify some (but not all) of those who go on to struggle. But it wouldn't be ethical to probe in this way, and this approach risks breaching the protection that individuals with mental health problems are entitled to under the law. Also when answering these questions, applicants would be prone to biasing their answers, just as they would with a questionnaire that asked directly about their emotional resilience. It's not the way forward.

But could these sorts of questions be asked *after* the selection process, in order to identify students who were likely to require additional emotional support? If the students knew that their responses would not be shared with the medical school faculty teaching them, they might be more likely to give honest answers. And then, if the students had been fully supported but still were unable to manage, faculty might find it easier to terminate a student's training. In other words, the 'failure to fail' tendency might be held in check.

*

Another email in my inbox. But this time it's from a colleague who has a senior training role in their particular specialty.

Had a really difficult day of annual reviews today. There just seem to be so many trainees with problems and I saw someone who is utterly failing ... Four years after leaving medical school, her supervisors said that she is barely functioning at medical student level. Anyway – I asked her about her under-graduate education. It won't surprise you to hear that she spent 12 years as a medical student because of repeated episodes of depression and anxiety ... I find that utterly unbelievable and completely depressing. How is such a thing possible? They have totally failed this trainee and the general public ... And all that it means is that she has invested several more years in a career that is going nowhere.

*

Medical schools need to acknowledge that the selection process doesn't (because it probably can't) provide a robust screening for emotional resilience. This means that, inevitably, there will be students in their institution who turn out not to be suited to the profession of medicine. I don't blame the institutions for selecting students who don't have what it takes to be a doctor because selection is, at best, an inexact science. But there is an urgent need to manage these students more effectively, once they start to struggle at medical school. Nobody should be allowed to train for a job for twelve years (and pay for that training) when there was no realistic prospect of success.

*

I decided to discuss my response to Kesia with my supervisor, Margaret. She's a clinical psychologist and psychotherapist and her perspective on my work is invaluable. I described how I had explained to Kesia that there is a legal framework in place that means she could not be discriminated against for health (including mental health reasons). In my email I had also told Kesia that the key issue was whether the illness would impact on her ability to get through the course and, following graduation, to work as a doctor. But this issue would be dealt with by occupational health, separately from the interview itself.

'Did you say anything else in your email?' Margaret asked.

I told Margaret about the different suggestions I had made to Kesia: that she should discuss her career intentions with the psychologists/psychiatrists treating her who were best placed to review whether now was a good time for her to apply; that she should try to get some relevant voluntary experience working with people who are sick, or frail or distressed, and ask herself how she found this sort of work; that she might want to give herself more time to get her anorexia under control and apply for medicine as a postgraduate; and that there were also careers in healthcare other than medicine that she might want to consider.

'And did you hear back?' Margaret asked.

'Yes, almost immediately. Kesia thanked me for taking the time to reply and said that she was considering other options, but her heart was still set on medicine.'

After this discussion with Margaret, I went back home and reread my email exchange with Kesia. I was struck by the fact that Kesia's email posed one question (Will the fact that I am still being treated for anorexia mean that I won't be allowed to study medicine?) whilst most of my email was actually devoted to answering something different. Kesia never explicitly asked for my opinion on whether she would be suited to medical training, given her long-standing anorexia. But that is the question I devoted most space to in my response.

Is it significant that Kesia didn't ask? Perhaps she was discussing her suitability for medical training with the clinical team treating her for anorexia. As I indicated in my email, they would be much better placed to have a view on this issue than I could ever be. But some of the doctors with eating disorders whom I have supported have been unable to face up to the impact of their illness on their capacity for medical work. And I'll never forget how one medical student with anorexia, who spent twelve years trying (but ultimately failing) to qualify, gave me an abridged career history in our first meeting. It was only after the session, when I matched her date of birth to her description of what had happened to her in medical school, that I realised that there was a gap of six years in her story. A gap that she couldn't bear to admit to me – even though she had come to see me in order to rebuild her career.

I contacted Kesia to ask if I could include her email in the chapter. Almost immediately she emailed me back, giving me permission, and updating me on what had happened:

> I did eventually apply to study medicine and have a place for next year. I was meant to be starting this October but unfortunately became unwell so had to defer the place. I am not ready to go anyway so I am concentrating on getting myself well enough to go next year.

For the time being, Kesia was on the receiving end of medical care, rather than training to be a doctor.

EPILOGUE

There's No Such Thing as a Doctor

If it wasn't for advances in medical science, my mother would have died when I was born. She was one of the first people in the UK to be successfully treated for a blood disorder – aplastic anaemia – which she developed towards the end of her pregnancy. As it was, her survival was far from guaranteed, during the first few weeks of my life. A quarter of a century later, my father developed myeloma – a cancer of the bone marrow. Although eventually he died from the disease, chemotherapy extended his life for over seven years.

The advances in medical science during the twentieth century, and continuing into the twenty-first, are extraordinary. Much of it we now take for granted; the vaccinations for diphtheria, tetanus and whooping cough – once childhood killers – that my grandchildren received when they were eight weeks old were only developed in the 1920s. The polio vaccine came later, in the 1950s. Ultrasound scans of the foetus were available when I had my children, but nowadays it is possible to perform surgical procedures on the foetus *in utero*.

Last year, a close friend in his early sixties with Primary Sclerosing Cholangitis – a relatively rare chronic liver disease – had a transplant. The donor was his 23-year-old son, who gifted his father 61% of his liver. Without the operation, this friend would have died of liver failure. The son has made a full recovery and my friend is doing well, although he will have to take immunosuppressant medication for life, to stop his own immune system rejecting his son's liver.

When I watch the video of the liver transplant operation (filmed with permission from my friend, as part of a series that the *Guardian* ran on the NHS), I am in awe. I remember talking to his wife on the day both her son and her husband were in hospital awaiting surgery. Her bravery was astonishing – I would have been in pieces. And the brief glimpses of the operation shown in the video increase my admiration for the surgical team a thousand-fold.

I am not a medical Luddite – somebody who turns their back on or scorns the achievements of 21st-century medicine. But there's an astonishing gap between, on the one hand, advances in medical practice and, on the other, our understanding of the psychological demands of medical work. It's almost as if the psyche has been surgically excised from our conception of what it means to be a doctor. In fact this psychic excision underpins all the stories in this book.

*

We've seen how doctors can have the intellectual ability to pass their medical school examinations but lack the psychological resilience to manage the emotional demands of medical work. We've also seen how the transition from medical student to junior hospital doctor represents a quantum shift in responsibility. And innovations such as the reduction in working hours that have been put in place to enhance junior doctors' well-being can have unforeseen psychological consequences when they erode the continuity of the clinical team.

We regularly require doctors to carry out extraordinarily distressing tasks with inadequate attention given to their psychological well-being. Then we blame doctors when their psychological defences kick in, and they respond to patients or relatives with a lack of empathy. Not only do we underestimate the emotional demands of clinical practice, but we also fail to recognise that some of the people who are attracted to the profession in the first place may be drawn to it out of a desire to manage their own psychological vulnerabilities. Clinicians' understanding of specialty choice is often woefully simplistic, with inadequate attention given to the psychological complexity embedded in the decision to treat a particular patient group.

Doctors can become ill or disabled, as can members of their family or close friends; inevitably, thoughts and feelings linked to the personal experience of illness will be evoked when doctors treat their patients. Medical work can involve sharing deeply private information as well as the exposure of intimate parts of the body. Doctors are not immune to developing sexual feelings for their patients but the training system denies that this could ever happen. The forces of sexism and racism that infect other professions are also found within medicine but the psychological impact of discrimination may be particularly devastating for doctors, given the enormous responsibility we require them to shoulder.

Even leaving the profession can be psychologically fraught. When doctors feel that they have been pushed to the edge, they frequently find themselves paralysed between equal, but opposing, forces. On the one hand, there is an enormous desire to leave medicine in order to escape from the psychological pressures of the work. On the other, there is terror that they might feel a failure, that they have let other people down, or that they may later wish they had stayed put. 'I'm just as scared that I may regret it if I stop,' was what Leo wrote in his email.

*

Taken together, doctors' psychological needs are denied, ignored, not thought about. Unmet. A systemic 'psycholectomy' has been performed on the profession as a whole. But its impact is felt most acutely in the doctor–patient relationship.

What is especially curious is that the psychological needs of one half of the dyad – the patient – are well recognised. So medical students and junior doctors are thoroughly versed in the mantra of 'patient-centred care'. They are taught and are tested on their communication skills and exhorted to show empathy to patients and family members. But if you dig a bit deeper, it soon becomes apparent that patient-centred care only tells half of the story. This becomes clearer if one makes a simple analogy with physics.

At secondary school I was taught the first law of thermodynamics. This law states that the energy within a system cannot be created or destroyed; it can only be transformed from one form to another. It strikes me that this basic law of physics has a psychic parallel. Perhaps it should be known as the first law of human dynamics? And just as the physical law demonstrates that the energy in a system cannot change but can only be transferred, the psychic law reminds us that a person's ability to carry out emotional work – to care for somebody else in distress – critically depends upon the quality of care that that person has themself received. It's almost as if the potential for giving care to others rests on a form of 'caring capital' that a person has accrued in the past. And currently. If a person feels uncared for, emotionally depleted, they will struggle (in some way or other) to carry the emotional burden of another person's suffering. They will struggle to care.

When it comes to the care of infants this basic principle is well understood. Mothers (and fathers) who are emotionally or physically depleted may struggle to provide effective and responsive care for their babies. And the emotional resources that a parent brings to bear – their caring capital – is influenced both by that parent's own experience of being parented in the past, as well as by their current networks of emotional support. None of this is controversial.

None of it is new, either. In the 1950s paediatrician and psychoanalyst Donald Winnicott wrote 'there is no such thing as a baby . . . a baby cannot exist alone, but is essentially part of a relationship'. I don't imagine that Winnicott would have been a proponent of 'infant-centred care'. He understood that the *relationship* between parent and child was all important.

Winnicott also recognised that the feelings that parents have for their children aren't always nice. In a classic paper, he lists eighteen reasons why a mother may, at times, experience hateful feelings towards her baby. These include:

He is ruthless, treats her as scum, an unpaid servant, a slave

His excited love is cupboard love, so that having got what he wants, he throws her away like orange peel

He is suspicious, refuses her good food, and makes her doubt herself, but eats well with his aunt

After an awful morning with him she goes out, and he smiles at a stranger, who says 'Isn't he sweet!'

Winnicott was playfully provocative in the way he framed these reasons – but at the same time he was highlighting a truth known to every parent. The palette of parental feelings doesn't only contain warm and sunny colours – it also spans murky, darker, hues. Of course, Winnicott wasn't advocating that parents should act out these feelings of hate; he was simply drawing attention to the inevitability of their existence. They are normal.

These two basic principles (the critical importance of the relationship between infant and parent, and the inevitability of hate alongside feelings of love towards one's baby) would be hard to dispute. But what is widely accepted in the context of mothers and babies is frequently overlooked when thinking about doctors and patients. Again this is extraordinary, because Winnicott explicitly made the parallel in the original paper when talking about the relationship between psychoanalysts and their patients.

*

Winnicott died in 1971. But if he were alive today, I wonder what reasons he would intuitively cite for doctors sometimes resenting, or even hating, their patients. Perhaps his list would include:

Fear of making a significant mistake

Time pressures; too many patients to see in too short a time

Uncertainty about the diagnosis, or treatment plan

Professional impotence when the patient's illness can't be cured

Patients' unrealistic expectations about what modern medicine can achieve

Patients challenging your professional knowledge

Fear of being the subject of a complaint or a legal claim

Exhaustion caused by working through the night

Hunger and thirst through working a whole shift without a break

Being on the receiving end of derogatory comments from patients

Disgust at physical decay or deformity

Fear of contagion

Contempt at injuries caused by the patient's own behaviour

Having to work in a part of the country where one is separated from family and friends

Missing out on a special family celebration because one has to work

And above all else, the reason why patients have always had, and will always have, the potential to evoke difficult feelings in the doctor is that inevitably they remind doctors that they, and those they love, are mortal.

*

Every item on the list is something that doctors have talked to me about over the years. The list isn't exhaustive but it illustrates the enormous psychological complexity of medical work. Of course, doctors are not the only ones who encounter these sorts of pressures. And other healthcare colleagues (for example nurses or midwives) have to put up with additional sources of stress such as low pay, or lack of recognition of their professional contribution. I've never forgotten old-style ward rounds where a busy nurse had to trundle behind the consultant for half the morning, yet was never once asked for her opinion on any of the patients under her care.

But it's the doctor who is responsible for diagnosing the illness, deciding on the best form of treatment, prescribing drugs, analysing progress and reviewing whether the treatment needs to be altered. Admittedly there are some senior nurses who, in certain contexts, take on some of these responsibilities. But from the fateful first Wednesday in August, junior doctors can be on call, running between different wards, tasked with making decisions which, if they get wrong, can have terrible consequences. Some doctors who come to see me cannot bear the nature of this responsibility. They agonise over the fact that a mistaken clinical decision could cost a life.

Doctors also have to cope with the sheer unpredictability and uncertainty of medical work. In medicine a given condition can present itself in a completely different way in two patients and whilst one may respond to a particular course of treatment, the other may not. This unpredictability weighs heavily on some doctors and is a frequent reason why so many of the doctors in this book have struggled.

*

One hundred and fifty years ago, the surgeon Joseph Lister published his findings on using antiseptics to reduce the risk of post-operative infections. Lister advocated the use of carbolic acid to disinfect the surgeon's hands, the instruments, the wound and even the air around the patient. When these simple measures were used, patient survival rates following amputation improved from 55% to 85%. But even with these extraordinary results, Lister's antiseptic methods were not immediately taken up by his colleagues; they found them complicated and time-consuming and tried to argue that the results were actually due to other changes such as improved ventilation in hospitals.

That was 1867. Today infection control informs every layer of medical practice: the GP washing their hands in their surgery after examining a patient; barrier nursing an immunosuppressed patient; isolating whole wards to control an outbreak of a hospital-acquired infection; and even national plans to manage the outbreak of a pandemic. In addition, many of the achievements of modern medicine are predicated on the capacity to control the spread of infection, and to treat it effectively when it occurs. Operations such as live-donor liver transplants wouldn't be possible if the risk of post-operative infection couldn't be minimised in both donor and host.

Just imagine, for a second, if the emotional well-being of the medical workforce (and the healthcare workforce more generally) was accorded the same priority as the control of infection. Parity between the infective, and the affective, in other words. In Lister's time, 45% of patients died of infection post-amputation. Today some reports suggest that over 50% of doctors experience burnout. Given this level of burnout (and of depression, and suicide) it would be hard to argue that we don't have a significant public health crisis on our hands. Is the comparison really so absurd?

The comparison also flags up that there's no one-off, simple solution. Infection control in a hospital isn't restricted to putting up a poster saying 'now wash your hands' in the toilets. Of course not. Yet I walked into the education centre of a London teaching hospital and saw a noticeboard covered in brick-patterned paper, at the top of which was the title 'resilience wall'. Staff members were encouraged to stick Post-it notes with upbeat comments ('I'll practise my breathing if I become stressed'; 'I'll go outside to get fresh air at lunchtime'). All good stuff, but the resilience wall is about as likely to have a serious impact on doctors' well-being as the brick-patterned paper is to bear the structural load of the building.

The problem with attempts to build doctors' resilience (and there have been many) is that they lay the blame at the foot of the individual. This approach is flawed, as the authors of a recent paper in the *BMJ* pointed out:

> Resilience is always contextual. It is a complex and dynamic
> interplay between an individual, the individual's environment and

sociocultural factors. Any intervention to promote resilience must deal with organisational as well as individual and team issues.

And that's what we've seen in this book. At the level of the individual, it's clear that some of the people who are selected into medicine are never going to be able to make it as doctors, that some doctors choose particular specialties out of an unconscious attempt to resolve their own personal conflicts, and that events going on in a doctor's private life can impact on how they feel about their work. These individual factors then interact with organisational ones – the systemic 'failure to fail'; the inverse-care law, in which those in greatest need of support end up receiving the least; the pressures of years of underfunding; the appalling lack of thought given to significant career transitions; the corrosive forces of sexism and racism, to name but a few. And the culture of medicine as a whole, with its reluctance to adopt an evidence-based approach to medical education and its tendency to disavow any signs of vulnerability on the part of the doctor and to lay blame at the foot of the individual is the glue loosely holding the system together.

Is it a wonder that there are cracks?

One thing is abundantly clear, and that is that there are no simple answers. Improving the emotional well-being of the medical workforce requires interventions that tackle all three interconnected levels – the individual, the organisation, and the culture of medicine as a whole.

It would be easy to despair, given the scale of the problem. But as we've seen in this book, across the world there are tiny flickers of hope. Michael Farquhar's sleep campaign needs to spread from London across the UK, and then to the rest of the world. It is a rare example of doctors using their clinical knowledge to benefit not only their patients – but also other clinicians. Many countries could learn from New Zealand and introduce a trainee intern year to manage the transition to clinical practice. Canada and the US are more enlightened than the UK when it comes to opening up medical training to those with physical disabilities, and the growth of the Schwartz Round movement across North America and the UK is encouraging. There are medical schools in the US that exemplify just what can be achieved when a commitment to diversity is tackled across an institution as a whole, while trainee doctors in the US would benefit from services like the Professional Support Unit where I worked in London.

Perhaps in 150 years' time, the attention given to doctors' emotional well-being will match that given currently to infection control. Perhaps historians looking back at how we treated doctors in 2018 will regard our medical systems with the same horror that we experience when we read about surgeons in Lister's day refusing to wash their hands between patients. Perhaps in 150 years' time, society will recognise that, whilst the demands of the job are exceptional, the person inhabiting the role of the doctor is, just like their patients, also human.

Perhaps.

NOTES

Introduction: Medicine in the Mirror

xxi   The Dean of the University wrote an impassioned opinion piece in the *New England Journal of Medicine*: Muller. D., 'Kathryn,' *N Engl J Med* 376 (2017), pp. 1101–1103.

xxi   The research the dean referred to is from the Mayo Clinic: Dyrbye, L. N., et al., 'Burnout and suicidal ideation among U.S. medical students,' *Ann Intern Med* 149 (2008), pp. 334–41.

The web page set up in Rose Polge's memory is available at: https://www.justgiving.com/teams/rosepolge.

The following year another junior doctor disappeared, and Dr Shaba Nabi wrote this article for *Pulse Today*, 31st March 2017: http://www.pulsetoday.co.uk/views/blogs/we-must-be-forced-to-care-for-ourselves/20034150.blog.

xxii   The 2016 study published in *The Lancet* concluded that GPs' clinical workload was reaching 'saturation point': Hobbs, R., et al., 'Clinical workload in UK primary care: A retrospective analysis of 100 million consultations in England, 2007–14,' *The Lancet* 387:4 (2016), pp. 2270–2272.

The quarterly monitoring report from The King's Fund is available online at: http://qmr.kingsfund.org.uk/2017/22/overview.

The survey of nearly 500 junior doctors conducted by the Royal College of Physicians reported that nearly 70% of doctors worked on a rota that was permanently under-staffed: Royal College of Physicians., 'Being a junior doctor: Experiences from the frontline of the NHS,' *RCP policy: workforce & Mission: Health* (2016) available online at: https://www.rcplondon.ac.uk/guidelines-policy/being-junior-doctor.

The 2016 GMC survey of junior doctors: GMC., 'National training survey 2016,' GMC (2016) available online at: https://www.gmc-uk.org/National_training_survey_2016___key_findings_68462938.pdf.

xxiii The following study carried out by researchers at Harvard Medical School reported that trainees who were suffering from depression made six times more medical errors than their non-depressed colleagues: Fahrenkopf, M. A., et al., 'Rates of medication errors among depressed and burnt out residents: prospective cohort study,' *BMJ* 336: 488 (2006), 10.1136/bmj.39469.763218.BE.

Wednesday's Child

7   The 2014 GMC conclusions on the August transition: Monrouxe, L. et al., 'UK Medical graduates preparedness for practice: Final report to the GMC,' *GMC* (2014) available online at: https://www.gmcuk.org/How_Prepared_are_UK_Medical_Graduates_for_Practice_SUBMITTED_Revised_140614.pdf_58034815.pdf

8   The Situational Judgement Test; example scenario taken from *SJT Answers & Rationale* available online at: http://www.foundation-programme.nhs.uk/pages/fp-afp/applicant-guidance/SJT/EPM.

10   Foundation Programme 2016 facts and statistics are available online at: http://www.foundationprogramme.nhs.uk/pages/resource-bank.

12   GP Julian Tudor-Hart's famously termed the 'inverse care' law in: Tudor-Hart, J., 'The inverse care law,' *The Lancet* 297: 7696 (1971), pp. 405–12.

13   For the 2016 data on Foundation Programme allocations see the *2016 UKFPO Annual Report* available online at: http://www.foundationprogramme.nhs.uk/news/story/annual-report-2016.

14   Information from the National Resident Matching Program available online at: http://www.nrmp.org/press-release-results-of-2016-nrmp-main-residency-match-largest-on-record-as-match-continues-to-grow/.

     Information on the algorithm that gained its two inventors a Nobel Prize in Economics is available online at: https://www.nobelprize.org/nobel_prizes/economic-sciences/laureates/2012/popular-economicsciences2012.pdf.

16   'April is the cruellest month' wrote Eliot in: 'The Waste Land', T. S. Eliot in *The Complete Poems and Plays of T.S. Eliot* (London: Faber and Faber, 1969).

     'Why July matters': Petrilli, M. C., et al., 'Why July matters,' *Acad Med* 91:7 (2016), pp. 910–912.

17   In 2009 a group of researchers at Imperial College London published this retrospective study: Jen, H. M., et al., 'Early in-hospitality mortality following trainee doctors' first day at work,' *PLoS ONE* 4:9 (2009), 10.1371/journal.pone.0007103.

18   In 2011, this research reported that 90% of physicians felt that the August transition had a negative impact on patient care: Vaughan, L., et al., 'August is always a nightmare: Results of the Royal College of Physicians Edinburgh and Society of acute medicine August transition survey,' *Clin Med* 11:4 (2011), pp. 322–6.

22   In 2014 the GMC found that the quality of induction was highly variable: Monrouxe, L., et al., 'UK Medical graduates preparedness for practice: Final report to the GMC,' GMC (2014) available

online at: https://www.gmc-uk.org/How_Prepared_are_UK_
Medical_Graduates_for_Practice_SUBMITTED_
Revised_140614.pdf_58034815.pdf.

25 Rose Polge's tragic suicide happened at the height of the junior
doctors' strike: Clarke, R., 'Suicides among junior doctors in the
NHS,' *BMJ* 357 (2017), 10.1136/bmj.j2527.

26 Psychologist Jenny Firth-Cozens' study of stress and depression
in junior doctors: Firth, J., 'Levels and source of stress in medical
students,' *Br Med J (Clin Res Ed)* 292 (1986), pp. 1177–80.

In 1987, Firth-Cozens reported the results of a longitudinal study
of first year junior doctors: Firth-Cozens, J., 'Emotional distress
in junior house officers,' *Br Med J (Clin Res Ed)* 295 (1987), pp.
533–6.

Twenty years after starting the first research project, Firth-Cozens
lamented that not enough had been done to support doctors'
wellbeing and stress: Firth-Cozens, J., 'Doctors, their wellbeing,
and their stress,' *BMJ* 326: 670 (2003), pp.670–671.

In 2015, this opinion piece was written following the suicide of
two first year residents: Goldman, L. M., et al., 'Depression and
suicide among physician trainees: Recommendations for a national
response,' *JAMA Psychiatry* 72:5 (2015), pp. 411–412.

A major international review of fifty-four studies in the *Journal
of the American Medical Association*: Mata, A. D., et al., 'Prevalence
of depression and depressive symptoms among resident physicians: A systematic review,' *JAMA* 314:22 (2015), pp. 2373–2383.

27 In an editorial accompanying the international review, the
authors concluded that personal and professional dysfunction
and suicide rate could be construed as a depression endemic
among residents: Schwenk, L. T., 'Resident depression. The tip
of a graduate medical education iceberg,' *JAMA* 314:22 (2015),
pp.2357–8.

28 This *BMJ* article, published in 1994, suggested that the New Zealand training model might have 'much to offer' the UK system: Allen, M. I. P., and Colls, M. B., 'Improving the preregistration experience: The New Zealand approach,' *BMJ* 308:6925 (1994), pp. 398–400.

29 The following survey from the *New Zealand Medical Journal* reported that at the end of the trainee intern year 92% of students felt prepared to be a doctor: Tweed, J. M., et al., 'How the trainee intern (TI) year can ease the transition from undergraduate education to postgraduate practice,' *N Z Med J* 123:1318 (2010), pp. 81–91.

Importantly, another study in New Zealand found that first year doctors' scored in the *normal* range for measures such as depression: Henning, A. M., et al., 'Junior doctors in their first year: mental health, quality of life, burnout and heart rate variability,' *Perspect Med Educ* 3:2 (2014), pp. 136–43.

30 A 2014 BMJ review found that limiting doctors' working hours reduced road traffic accidents caused by exhausted doctors: Rodriguez-Jarneo, C. M., et al., 'European working time directive and doctors' health: a systematic review of the available epidemiological evidence,' *BMJ Open* 4 (2014), 10.1136/bmjopen-2014-004916.

31 Reducing working hours does not reduce fatigue as one trainee commented in: Morrow, G., et al., 'Have restricted working hours reduced junior doctors' experience of fatigue?' A focus group and telephone interview study. *BMJ Open* 4 (2014), 10.1136/bmjopen-2013-004222.

Michael Farquhar's piece in the *BMJ* 'We must recognise the health effects associated with shift working,' available online at http://blogs.bmj.com/bmj/2017/10/06/michael-farquhar-we-must-recognise-the-health-effects-associated-with-shift-working/.

32   Details about the HALT campaign can be found online at: http://
      www.kingshealthpartners.org/latest/1028-staff-encouraged-to-
      take-regular-breaks.

33   The GMC annual trainee survey found that more than 50% of
      doctors in training worked beyond their rostered hours: 'National
      training survey 2016: Key findings,' GMC (2016) available
      online at: https://www.gmc-uk.org/National_training_survey_
      2016___key_findings_68462938.pdf.
      The British government review, commissioned by the Secretary
      of State for Health, reviewed the impact of the European Time
      Directive on the quality of training: Temple, J., 'Time for training:
      A review of the impact of the European Time Directive on the
      quality of training,' (2010) available online at: https://www.hee.
      nhs.uk/sites/default/files/documents/Time%20for%20
      training%20report_0.pdf.

34   There is some evidence that more recent groups of trainees
      welcome restrictions on working hours: Morrow, G., et al., 'The
      impact of the Working Time regulations on medical education
      and training: Literature Review, a report for the General Medical
      Council,' *Centre for Medical Education Research, Durham
      University* (2012).
      Female trainees have been found to be more positive about
      working hour restrictions than their male counterparts: Maybury,
      C.; 'The European Working Time Directive: a decade on,' *The
      Lancet* 384:9954 (2014), pp. 1562–1563.

35   Psychiatrist Gwen Adshead's article in *Medical Education*:
      Adshead, G., 'Becoming a caregiver: attachment theory and poorly
      performing doctors,' *Med Edu* 44:2 (2010) pp. 125–31.
      The Libby Zion case in: Patel, N., 'Learning lessons: The Libby
      Zion case revisited', *Journal of the American College of Cardiolog*
      64:25 (2014), pp. 2802–4.

36 Resident duty hours across the globe in: Temple, J., 'Resident duty hours around the globe: where are we now?' *BMC Med Educ* 14 (Suppl 1): S8 (2014).
A systematic review of 135 studies on the impact of duty hour restrictions: Ahmed, N., et al., 'A systematic review of the effects of resident duty hour restrictions in surgery,' *Ann Surg* 259:6 (2014), pp. 1041–53.

Finding the Middle

49 Paediatrician and psychoanalyst John Bowlby studied the psychological bonds that develop between infants and carers: Bowlby, J., 'Separation Anxiety,' *International Journal of Psycho-Analysis* 41 (1959); Bowlby, J., *Attachment and Loss, Vol.1: Attachment* (London: Hogarth Press and Institute of Psycho-Analysis, 1969); Bowlby, J., *Attachment and Loss, Vol.2: Separation: Anxiety and Anger* (London: Hogarth Press and Institute of Psycho-Analysis, 1973); Bowlby, J., *Attachment and Loss, Vol.3: Loss: Sadness and Depression* (London: Hogarth and Press and Institute of Psycho-Analysis, 1980).

50 Bowlby's student, Dr Mary Ainsworth, conducted a series of observational experiments to assess differences in how infants were attached to their parents, see: Farnfield, S., and Holmes, P., eds., *The Routledge Handbook of Attachment: Assessment* (London and New York: Routledge, 2014).

51 The identification of 'disorganized' attachment: Main, M., and Solomon, J., 'Discovery of an insecure – disorganized / disoriented attachment pattern,' in Brazelton, B., and Yogman, W. M., eds., *Affective Development in Infancy* (New Jersey: Ablex, 1986). The Adult Attachment Interview: Hesse, E., 'The Adult Attachment Interview: Protocol, method of analysis and empirical studies,' in

Cassidy, J., and Shaver, P. R., eds., *Handbook of Attachment: Theory, research and clinical applications, 2nd ed.,* (New York: McGraw Hill, 2008).

52   Patients who regularly go to their GP with vague, undiagnosed medical symptoms tend to have insecure attachment styles: Taylor, R. E., et al., 'Insecure attachment and frequent attendance in primary care: a longitudinal cohort study of medically unexplained symptom presentations in ten UK general practices,' *Psychol Med* 42:4 (2012), pp. 855–64.

The following researchers found that terminally ill cancer patients, with a secure attachment style, had a greater capacity to form a close working alliance with their physician: Vincenzo, C., et al., 'Reciprocal empathy and working alliance in terminal oncological illness: The Crucial Role of Patients Attachment Style,' *J Psychosoc Oncol* 32:5 (2014), pp. 517–34.

Gwen Adshead's description in: Adshead, G., 'Becoming a caregiver: attachment theory and poorly performing doctors,' *Med Educ* 44:2 (2010), pp. 125–31.

56   George Vaillant's mechanisms of defense in: Vaillant, G., *Adaptation to Life* (Cambridge: Harvard University Press, 1977).

57   Psychiatrist and social anthropologist, Simon Sinclair's *Making Doctors*: Sinclair, S., *Making Doctors: An institutional apprenticeship* (Oxford: Berg Publishers, 1997).

58   Danielle Ofri described the experience of a paediatric trainee in: Ofri, D., *What Doctors Feel* (Boston: Beacon Press, 2013).

A recent systematic review concluded a consistent decline in empathy as training progressed: Neumann, M., et al., 'Empathy decline and its reasons: A systematic review of studies with medical students and residents,' *Acad Med* 86:8 (2011), pp. 996–1009.

59   William Osler's essay *Aequanimitas in*: Osler, W., *Aequanimitas* (New York: Norton, 1963).

Renee Fox and psychiatrist Harold Leif's 'detached concern' in: Fox, R., and Leif, H., 'Training for "Detached Concern" in Medical Students,' in Harold, I., Leif, V., et al., eds., *The Psychological basis of Medical Practice* (New York: Harper and Row, 1963).

The statement produced by the Society for General Internal Medicine on empathy: Markais, K., et al., 'Teaching empathy: It can be done,' *Working paper presented at the Annual Meeting of the Society of General Internal Medicine in San Francisco, April 29 – May 1, (1999).*

60   Psychiatrist Jodi Halpern's research on detachment and a doctor's effectiveness in: Halpern, J., 'Clinical Empathy in Medical Care,' in Decety, J., ed., *Empathy: from bench to bedside* (Massachusetts Institute of Technology: MIT Press, 2014).

A study of over 7,000 physicians found that those with great empathic concern for their patients were more satisfied with their work: Gleichgerrcht, E., and Decety, J., 'Empathy in clinical practice: How individual dispositions, gender, and experience moderate empathic concern, burnout and emotional distress in physicians,' *PLoS ONE* 8:4 (2013), 10.1371/journal.pone.0061526.

Michael Crichton's description of human dissection in: Crichton, M., *Travels* (New York: Vintage Books, 2014).

61   Kenneth Schwartz wrote about his experience of being a patient for the *Boston Globe Magazine* in: Schwartz, B. K., 'A patient's story,' *Boston Globe* (July 16th, 1995) available online at: https://www.bostonglobe.com/magazine.

62   The *Schwartz Center Rounds* are described in: Penson, T. R., et al., 'Connection: Schwartz Center Rounds at Massachusetts General Hospital cancer centre,' *Oncologist* 15:7 (2010), pp. 760–764.

Information on the adoption of *Schwartz Center Rounds* is available online at www.theschwartzcenter.org.

63   The *BMJ* argued, 'we do not know what proportion of staff ...
      may need to attend (Schwartz) Rounds' in: Robert, G., et al.,
      'Exploring the adoption of Schwartz Center Rounds as an organ-
      isational innovation to improve staff well-being in England, 2009
      – 2014,' *BMJ Open* 7 (2017), 10.1136/bmjopen-2016-014326.
      Staff comments on using Schwartz Centre Rounds in this 2017
      study: Farr, M., and Barker, R., 'Can staff be supported to deliver
      compassionate care through implementing Schwartz Rounds in
      community and mental health services?' *Qual Health Res* 27:11
      (2017), pp. 1652–1663.

72   Research from the King's Fund highlighted that enabling students
      to hear patients personal experience of care is effective in
      enhancing compassion: Firth-Cozens, J., and Cornwell, J., 'The
      Point of Care: Enabling compassionate care in acute hospital
      settings' (2009), available online at https://www.kingsfund.org.
      uk/publications/articles/enabling-compassionate-care-acute-
      hospital-settings.

Which Doctor

81   John Ballatt and Penelope Campling described how the uncon-
      scious motivation to heal can become channelled into a relentless
      drive to work, in their book: Ballatt, J., and Campling, P.,
      Intelligent Kindness: Reforming the culture of healthcare (London:
      Royal College of Psychiatrists, 2011).

88   In 2014 the World Psychiatric Association (WPA) study found
      evidence between personal experience of mental illness and
      choosing to specialize in psychiatry: Farooq, K., et al., 'Why
      medical students choose psychiatry – a 20 country cross-
      sectional survey,' *BMC Med Educ* 14:12 (2014), 10.1186/1472-
      6920-14-12.

89 Dr Mike Shooter's description of his own struggles with depression in: Shooter, M., 'Depression,' *BMJ* 326 (2003), pp. 1324–5. The notion that a doctor's capacity stems from their own suffering has ancient roots, for example, *Plato's Republic*. Quoted in Jackson, W. S., 'Presidential Address: The Wounded Healer,' *Bull Hist Med* 75: 1 (2001), pp. 1–36.

90 In contemporary psychotherapeutic practice, the idea of the 'wounded healer' is closely associated with the writings of Carl Jung: Jung, C., *The practice of psychotherapy: Essays on the psychology of the transference of other subjects* ([trans. RFC Hull] NJ: Princeton University Press, 1966).

The link between personal experience of mental illness and wanting to help others who have similar conditions applies to psychologists and psychotherapists: Ivey, G., and Partington, T., 'Psychological woundedness and its evaluation in applications for clinical psychological training,' *Clin Psychol Psychother* 21: 2 (2014), pp. 166–77.

92 In the UK doctors have the choice of sixty-six specialties. Further information is available online at: https://www.gmc-uk.org/education/approved_curricula_systems.asp.

Information on the thirty-seven specialties on offer in the US is available online at: http://www.abms.org/.

Information on the eighty-five specialties on offer in Australia is available online at: http://www.medicalboard.gov.au/.

The following 2013 survey of over 7,000 doctors in the States found that between a third and a quarter were not happy with the specialties that they had chosen: Liselott, N. D., et al., 'Physician satisfaction and burnout at different career stages,' *Mayo Clinic Proceedings* 88:12 (2013), pp. 1358–1367.

Nearly 20% of oncology and surgical trainees in the States would not choose their specialty again: Shanafelt, D. T., et al., 'Oncology fellows' career plans, expectations and well-being: Do fellows know what they are getting into?' *J Clin Oncol* 32:27 (2014), pp. 2991–7; Tchantchaleishvili, V., et al., 'Current integrated cardiothoracic surgery residents: a thoracic surgery association survey,' *Ann Thorac Surg* 99:3 (2015), pp. 1040–7.

In a UK study, 34% of obstetric trainees regretted their specialty choice: Thangaratinam, S., et al., 'Specialist training in obstetrics and gynaecology: a survey on work-life balance and stress among trainees in UK,' *J Obstet Gynaecol* 26:4 (2006), pp. 302–4.

93   In the States this study found that over 94% of anaesthetists were satisfied that they had chosen the right career: Augustin, I. D., et al., 'Recruitment of house staff into anesthesiology: a longitudinal evaluation of factors for selecting a career in anesthesiology and an individual training program,' *J Clin Anesth* 26:2 (2014), pp. 91–105. Dissatisfaction is contagious: Liselott, N. D., et al., 'Physician satisfaction and burnout at different career stages,' *Mayo Clinic Proceedings* 88:12 (2013), pp. 1358–1367.

Harvard researchers compared the personalities of medical and surgical trainees using the Rorschach inkblot test: Stanley, H., et al., 'The surgical personality: A comparison of medical and surgical residents with the Rorschach,' *Cardiovasc Dis* 2:2 (1975), pp. 117–128.

94   This review, in a leading psychological journal, concluded that the Rorschach method is reliable: Kivisalu, T. M., et al., 'An investigation of interrater for the Rorschach Performance System (R-PAS) in a nonpatient U.S. sample,' *J Pers Assess* (2016), pp. 1–9.

There are studies that have used standardized personality questionnaires that agree with the Harvard findings, for example: Warschkow, R., et al., 'A comparative cross-sectional study of personality traits in internists and surgeons,' *Surgery* 148:5 (2010), pp. 901–7.

Some studies have found that surgeons are more extravert than doctors in other specialties, for example: MacNeily, E. A., et al., 'The surgical personality: comparisons between urologists, non-urologists and non-surgeons,' *Can Urol Assoc J* 5:3 (2011), pp. 182–85.

Some studies have also found that surgeons are less warm and considerate compared to doctors in other specialties, for example: Bexelius, T. S., et al., 'Association between personality traits and future choice of specialization among Swedish doctors: a cross-sectional study,' *Postgrad Med J* 92 (2016), pp. 441–446.

95   A selection of studies on role models: Ravindra, P., and Fitzgerald, E. J., 'Defining surgical role models and their influence on career choice,' *World Journal of Surgery* 35: 4 (2011), pp. 704–9; Murinson, B. B., et al., 'Formative experiences of emerging physicians: gauging the impact of events that occur during medical school,' *Acad Med* 85:8 (2010), pp. 1331–7; Stahn, B., and Harendza, S., 'Role models play the greatest role – a qualitative study on reasons for choosing postgraduate training at a university hospital,' *GMS Z Med Ausbild* 31:4 (2014), Doc45.

96   The Medical Education paper 'Trying on Possible Selves': Burack, J. H., et al., 'A study of medical students' specialty-choice pathways: trying on possible selves,' *Acad Med* 72:6 (1997), pp. 534–41. A selection of studies have found that medical students and junior doctors tend to choose specialties that they have enjoyed in medical school and the early years of clinical practice: Maisonneuve, J. J., et al., 'Career choices for geriatric medicine: national surveys of graduates of 1974–2009 all UK medical schools,' *Age Aging* 43:4 (2014), pp. 535–541; Smith, F., et al., 'Factors influencing junior doctors' choices of future specialty: trends over time and demographics based on results from UK national surveys,' *J R Soc Med* 108:10 (2015), pp. 396–405.

99 Findings from researchers in Oxford, on specialty choice and work-life balance: Smith, F., et al., 'Factors influencing junior doctors' choices of future specialty: trends over time and demographics based on results from UK national surveys,' *J R Soc Med* 108:10 (2015), pp. 396–405.

100 In the States, the director of Medical Education observed that 'millennials seem to be more inclined to trade some of their income for more control of their hours' in: Glicksman, E., 'Wanting it all: a new generation of doctors' places higher value on work-life balance,' *AAMC Reporter* (2013) available online at: https://www.aamc.org/newsroom/reporter/336402/work-life.html.

Studies in Australia and Canada have also found that doctors place a higher value on work-life balance than previous generations: Tolhurst, H. M., and Stewart, A. M., 'Balancing work, family and other lifestyle aspects: a qualitative study of Australian medical students' attitudes,' *Med J Aust* 181:7 (2004), pp. 361–4; Results from the 2010 National Physician Survey in Canada available online at: http://nationalphysiciansurvey.ca/wp-content/uploads/2012/05/NPS2010-Students-Binder.pdf.

101 A 2015 study of over 15,000 doctors found that student debt had influenced specialty choice: Smith, F., et al., 'Factors influencing junior doctors' choices of future specialty: trends over time and demographics based on results from UK national surveys,' *J R Soc Med* 108:10 (2015), pp. 396–40.

In the US, the median indebtedness at graduation for medical students was $170,000: Rohlfing, J., et al., 'Medical student debt and major life choices other than specialty,' *Med Educ Online* 19 (2014), 10.3402/meo.v19.25603.

Students with higher debt were more likely to choose a specialty with a higher average annual income, as found by: Rohlfing

J., et al., 'Medical student debt and major life choices other than specialty,' *Med Educ Online* 19 (2014), 10.3402/meo.v19.25603. Increasing financial debt has been found to correlate with students' reports of depression, for example: Mader, M. E., et al., 'The temporal decline of idealism in two cohorts of medical students at one institution,' *BMC Med Educ* 14:58 (2014), 10.1186/1472–6920-14-58.

108   In the following article, psychologist Tom Kreishok argues that rationality has its limits: Krieshok, S. T., et al., 'Career decision making: The limits of rationality and the abundance of non-conscious processes,' *J Vocat Behav* 75 (2009), pp. 275–290.

Brief Encounter

111   A study published in 2015 found that over a quarter of medical students in the US and Canada who identified themselves as belonging to a minority sexual orientation concealed this in medical school: Mansh, M., et al., 'Sexual and gender minority identity disclosure during undergraduate medical education: "In the Closet" in medical school,' *Acad Med* 90:5 (2015), pp. 634–44.

115   Freud's notion of transference in: Freud, S., *Introductory lectures on psychoanalysis*, se., XV – XVI (1916–1917 [1915–1917]).

119   In 1997, Kapsalis wrote of the precarious relationship between pelvic exams and sex acts in a detailed study of how doctors are taught gynaecology: Kapsalis, T., *Public privates: Performing gynaecology from both ends of the speculum* (Durham and London: Duke University Press, 1997).

120   As an example, Kapsalis quoted a male physician in: Kapsalis, T., *Public privates: Performing gynaecology from both ends of the speculum* (Durham and London: Duke University Press, 1997).

A major review of the teaching of pelvic examinations concluded that the 'psychological impact' on the learner was not well explored in the literature: Jha, V., et al., 'Patient involvement in teaching and assessing intimate examination skills: a systematic review', *Med Educ* 44:4 (2010), pp. 347–57.

Since the late 1970s, the issue of consent around the intimate examination of anaesthetised female patients has been widely debated: Ralph, W., et al., 'Professional patients: An improved method of teaching breast and pelvic examination,' *J Reprod Med* 19:3 (1977), pp.163–6; Holzman, G. B., et al., 'Initial pelvic examination instructions: The effectiveness of three contemporary approaches,' *Am J Obstet Gynecol* 129:2 (1977), pp. 124–9; Robertson, N., 'Panel faults, breast, pelvic test methods,' *New York Times* (1969).

121   Recent patient surveys indicate that attitudes of the general public have moved on, with women expecting to be asked before medical students practise intimate examinations on them: Wainberg, S., 'Teaching pelvic examinations under anaesthesia: what do women think?' *J Obstet Gynaecol Can* 32:1 (2010), pp. 49–53.

A survey published in 2011 found that students still find themselves in situations where they are asked to conduct intimate examinations without asking the patients: Rees, C., and Monrouxe, R., 'Medical students learning intimate examinations without valid consent: a multicentre study,' *Med Educ* 45 (2011), pp. 261–72.

'This article is dangerous', a counter-argument from: Kaushik, N., 'Please don't touch me there: the ethics of intimate examinations. What examination is not intimate?' *BMJ* 326:1326 (2003), 10.1136/bmj.326.7402.1326-b. In response to: Coldicott, Y., et al., 'The ethics of intimate examinations – teaching tomorrow's doctors,' *BMJ* 326:7380 (2003), pp.97–101, an article from th *BMJ* about the need to gain informed consent.

122 In 2009, the article titled 'The other side of the speculum' caused fury online: Thoma, B., 'The other side of the speculum,' *Can Fam Physician* 55:11 (2009) p. 1112; Pimlott, N., et al., 'Uncomfortable reflections,' *Can Fam Physician* 56:3 (2010), pp. 221–222.

In response to the 'The other side of the speculum': Andres, E. D., 'The other side of the spectrum,' *Can Fam Physician* 56:3 (2010) p. 221.

American psychiatrist Julius Buchwald wrote of students' first pelvic examination in: Buchwald, J., 'The first pelvic examination: Helping students cope with their emotional reactions,' *J Med Educ* 54:9 (1979) pp. 725–8.

123 The following 2014 Australian study found students used jokes when uncomfortable sexual feelings were discussed: Dabson, M. A., et al., 'Medical students' experiences learning intimate physical examination skills: a qualitative study,' *BMC Med Educ* 14:39 (2014), 10.1186/1472–6920-14–39.

Freud, in his *Jokes and Their Relation to the Unconscious* was first to explore how jokes bear the traces of repressed desire: Freud, S., *Jokes and Their Relation to the Unconscious* (Harmondsworth: Penguin [Original work published in 1905]).

124 Balint groups were started in London in the 1950s: Balint, M., and Balint, E., *The doctor his patient and the illness*, 2nd ed., (London: Pitman Medical, 1968).

125 As one participant explained: 'you leave the group relieved ...' in: Steinlieb, J. L; Scott, P; Lichtenstein, A., Nease, D. E and Freedy, J. R., 'Balint Group Process: Optimizing the Doctor-Patient Relationship,' in O'Reilly-Landry, M., ed., *A psychodynamic understanding of Modern Medicine: Placing the person at the center of Care* (London: Radcliffe Publishing, 2012).

127 The GMC guidelines on: 'Maintaining a professional relationship between you and your patient,' *GMC online* (2013) available online at: https://www.gmc-uk.org/guidance/ethical_guidance.

128 The Medical Council of New Zealand's guidance on professional boundaries: 'Sexual boundaries in the doctor-patient relationship: A resource for doctors,' available online at: https://www.mcnz.org.

The GMC failed to incorporate the findings of a national research project on sexual boundary violations in healthcare: Halter, M., et al., 'Sexual Boundary Violations by Health Professionals – an overview of the published empirical literature,' *CHRE* (2007); CHRE: 'Clear sexual boundaries between healthcare professionals and patients: responsibilities of healthcare professionals,' *CHRE* (2008) both are available online via: https://www.professional-standards.org.uk.

135 Horsfall, S., 'Doctors who commit suicide while under GMC fitness to practice investigation. Internal review,' *GMC online* (2014) available online at: https://www.gmc-uk.org/Internal_review_into_suicide_in_FTP_processes.pdf_59088696.pdf.

Role Reversal

143 The extreme difficulty of being both a doctor and a patient in: Klitzman, R., *When Doctors Become Patients* (New York: Oxford University Press, 2008).

149 The author Michael Crichton and his comments on the role of human dissection in: Crichton, M., *Travels* (New York: Vintage Books, 2004).

Two researchers concluded that dissection 'has the effect of setting the medical student apart from others' in: Madill, A., and Latchford, G., 'Identity change and the human dissection expe▪

ence over the first year of medical training,' *Soc Sci Med* 60 (2005), pp. 1637–1647.

Psychiatrist and psychoanalyst Norman Straker's experience as a medical student as described in: Straker, N., ed., *Facing Cancer and the Fear of Death: A Psychoanalytic Perspective on Treatment.* (Lanham Maryland: Jason Aronson, 2012).

150 Sabine Hildebrandt's strategies for the anatomy curriculum: Hildebrandt, S., 'Thoughts on practical core elements of an ethical anatomical education,' *Clin Anat* 29 (2016), pp.37–45.

Some medical schools have abandoned the use of human dissection as a way of teaching anatomy: Patel, B. S., et al., 'Is dissection the only way to learn anatomy? Thoughts from students at a non-dissecting medical school,' *Perspect Med Educ* 4 (2015), pp. 259–260. In medical schools that use human dissection, the cadaver is still routinely referred to as the 'first patient': Bohl, M., et al., 'Medical students' perceptions of the body donor as a 'first patient' or 'teacher': a pilot study,' *Anat Sci Educ* 4:4 (2011), pp. 208–13.

155 Julie Madorsky, a physical medicine and rehabilitation specialist, wrote of her teaching experiences in: Corbet, B., and Madorsky, J., 'Physicians with disabilities,' *West J Med* 154 (1991), pp. 514–521.

156 Thoughtlessness, with regards to disabled access, has been detailed in studies such as: Steinberg, G. A., et al., 'Reasonable accommodations for medical faculty with disabilities,' *JAMA* 288: 24 (2002), pp. 3147–54.

A doctor who walked with crutches described his experience of attending an interview for an academic position in: Steinberg, G. A., et al., 'Reasonable accommodations for medical faculty with disabilities,' *JAMA* 288: 24 (2002), pp. 3147–54.

A doctor who relied on crutches described her first hospital post as 'an environment of isolation': Corbet, B., and Madorsky, J., 'Physicians with disabilities,' *West J Med* 154 (1991), pp.514–521.

157   Jenny Morris writing on disability in: Watermeyer, B., 'Disability
      and Psychoanalysis,' in Watermeyer, B., Swartz, L., Lorenzo, T.,
      et al., eds. *Disability and Social Change: A South African Agenda*
      (Cape Town: HSRC Press, 2006).
      The report by the BMA Equal Opportunities Committee in 2007
      is available online at: http://www.hscbusiness.hscni.net/pdf/
      BMA_Disability_equality_in_the_medical_profession_
      July_2007_pdf.
      A 2009 study, in a Scottish medical school, found that there was
      a great deal of under-reporting of impairment by doctors: Miller,
      S., et al., 'Medical students' attitudes towards disability and
      support for disability in medicine,' *Med Teach* 31 (2009), pp.
      556–561.
      Some medical schools have introduced a 'card' scheme to
      empower students with disabilities or health conditions: Cook,
      V., et al., 'Supporting students with disability and health issues:
      lowering the social barriers,' *Med Educ* 46 (2012), pp. 564–574.

158   The UK Equality Act 2010, available online at: https://www.
      equalityhumanrights.com/en/equality-act/equality-act-2010.
      The Americans with Disabilities Act of 1990, available online at:
      https://www.ada.gov/ada_intro.htm.

159   The GMC major review of health and disability in medical educa-
      tion and training is available online at: https://www.gmc-uk.
      org/H_26D_review_statement___May_13.pdf_56450036.pdf.

160   A GMC publication entitled 'Achieving Good Medical Practice:
      A Guide for Medical Students' available online at: https://www.
      gmc-uk.org/Achieving_good_medical_practice_0816.
      pdf_66086678.pdf.pdf.

161   Jemma Saville's article 'Guidance for disabled students,' (April
      2008) is available online at: http://careers.bmj.com/careers
      advice/view-article.html?id=2897.

Jemma Saville's story was included in a BMA publication entitled 'A Celebration of Disabled Doctors,' (December 2009) and is available online at: http://www.hscbusiness.hscni.net/pdf/BMA-_Disabled_doctors_December_2009_pdf.pdf.

162 Jemma Saville's petition page: 'Petition for partially sighted doctor to be allowed to practise,' available at: http://www.thepetitionsite.com/1/help-VI-doctor/.

163 Tim Cordes' description of how he managed to complete his medical degree: Cordes, T., 'A practicing blind physician,' *Braille Monitor* 53:10 (2010).

164 Dr Dean Krahn described Tim Cordes' treatment of veterans with addiction problems in the article 'Blind doc at VA sees patients differently,' (June 2013). The article is available online at: https://www.va.gov/health/NewsFeatures/2013/June/Blind-Doc-at-VA-Sees-Patients-Differently.asp.

165 Clinical psychologist Brian Watermeyer wrote 'disabled people remain unknown' in Watermeyer, B., *Towards a Contextual Psychology of Disablism* (London: Routledge, 2013).

166 Canadian doctor, Jessica Dunkley is one of the first deaf doctors in the country: Moulton, D., 'Physicians with disabilities often undervalued,' *CMAJ* 189:18 (2017), e678-e679.

Leaky Pipes

174 Isobel Allen's study of women doctors: Allen, I., *Doctors and their careers*, 1st ed., (London: Policy Studies Institute, 1988).
The National Working Group on Women in Medicine report, 'Women doctors: making a difference' is available online at: https://hee.nhs.uk/sites/default/files/documents/WIMreport.pdf.

75 A study published in the *BMJ* in 2016 reported negative attitudes towards pregnancy and maternity/paternity leave: Rich, A., et al.,

'You can't be a person and a doctor: the work–life balance of doctors in training—a qualitative study,' *BMJ Open*, 6:12 (2016), 10.1136/bmjopen-2016–013897.

176 Social anthropologist Joan Cassell's study in: Cassell, J., *The woman in the surgeon's body* (Cambridge, Mass: Harvard University Press, 1998).

179 A study published in the *American Journal of Surgery* in 2016 found that half of the women in the study felt discriminated against based on their gender: Seemann, N., et al., 'Women in academic surgery: why is the playing field still not level?' *Am J Surg* 211: 2 (2016), pp. 343–349.

A 2016 study published in the *British Medical Journal* reported responses from trainee female surgeons: Rich, A., et al., 'You can't be a person and a doctor: the work–life balance of doctors in training—a qualitative study,' *BMJ Open* 6:12 (2016), 10.1136/bmjopen-2016–013897.

180 According to Jyoti Shah, a consultant urological surgeon in the UK, female surgeons still encounter comments on menstruation in the operating theatre: Harley, N., 'Sexism in surgery: Females being put off becoming surgeons by men,' *Telegraph* available online at: http://www.telegraph.co.uk/news/health/11903476/Sexism-in-surgery-Females-being-put-off-becoming-surgeons-by-men.html.

In 1863 Elizabeth Garrett Anderson wrote to the Aberdeen Medical School, requesting permission to attend classes: Anderson, L., *Elizabeth Garrett Anderson 1836–1917* (Cambridge: Cambridge University Press, [reprint] 2016).

181 Canadian physician William Osler in: Moldow, G., *Women doctors in gilded-age Washington* 1st ed., (Urbana and Chicago: University of Illinois Press, 1987).

182 By the end of the Second World War, 25% of medical students were female, although after the war, ex-servicemen returned t

claim university places: Pringle, R., *Sex and Medicine. Gender, power and authority in the medical profession* (Cambridge: Cambridge University Press, 1998).

In 1962, just over 20% of UK medical students were women. Twenty years later the proportion rose to 45.3%. Figures available online at: https://www.gov.uk/government/uploads/system/uploads/attachment_data/file/507651/CfWI_future_consultant_workforce.pdf.

Latest figures for the UK show that 55% of medical students are women. Figures available online at: http://www.gmc-uk.org/SOMEP_2013_web.pdf_53703867.pdf.

Between 1970 and 1980, the proportion of female medical students more than doubled: Walsh, M. R., 'The rediscovery of the need for a feminist medical education,' *Harv Educ Rev* 49:4 (1979), pp. 447–466.

The latest US figures, for 2016 entry, indicate that, for the first time, parity has almost been achieved: News.aamc.org., 'Number of Female Medical School Enrollees Reaches 10-Year High,' available online at: https://news.aamc.org/press-releases/article/applicant-enrollment-2016/.

184   Female GPs tend to have a significantly higher proportion of lengthy consultations than their male counterparts: Hedden, L., et al., 'The implications of the feminization of the primary care physician workforce on service supply: a systematic review,' *Hum Resour Health* 12:32 (2014), 10.1186/1478-4491-12-32.

185   A 2015 study of over 15,000 doctors: Lambert, T. W., et al., 'Trends in attractiveness of general practice as a career: surveys of views of UK-trained doctors,' *Br J Gen Pract* 67:657 (2017), 10.3399/bjgp17X689893.

186   The proportion of female consultants in obstetrics/gynaecology in the UK in: 'State of Medical Education and Practice,' GMC

(2016) available online at: https://www.gmc-uk.org/SoMEP_2016_Overview.pdf_68137053.pdf.

187   A 2016 survey of over 10,000 doctors in the UK found that 42% of women worked part time: Lachish, S., et al., 'Factors associated with less-than-full-time working in medical practice: results of surveys of five cohorts of UK doctors, 10 years after graduation,' *Hum Resour Health*, 14:1 (2016), 10.1186/s12960-016-0162-3.

188   Perhaps most shocking of all, women doctors are paid less than their male counterparts: Connolly, S., and Holdcroft, A., 'The Pay Gap for Women in Medicine and Academic Medicine,' BMA (2009) available online at: http://www.medicalwomensfederation.org.uk/images/Daonload_Pay_Gap_Report.pdf.

Salary discrepancies have also been reported in the States: Willett, L., et al., 'Gender Differences in Salary of Internal Medicine Residency Directors: A National Survey,' *Am J Med*, 128:6 (2016), pp. 659–665.

Sir Liam Donaldson in the 'Report of the Chair of the National Working Group on Women in Medicine,' (2009) available online at: https://hee.nhs.uk/sites/default/files/documents/WIMreport.pdf.

191   Responses from the BMA 2009 report available online at: http://www.medicalwomensfederation.org.uk/images/Daonload_Pay_Gap_Report.pdf.

Studies from the US are replete with horror stories that women faced when they attempted to continue training with a young family: Boulis, A., and Jacobs, J., *The Changing Face of Medicine: Women Doctors and the Evolution of Health Care in America* (Ithaca and London: Cornell University Press, 2008).

196   'Ladies would make bad doctors, at best': Anderson, L., *Elizabeth Garrett Anderson 1836–1917* (Cambridge: Cambridge Universit Press, [reprint] 2016).

A 2017 study published in the Journal of the American Medical Association found that sick older patients did better if the doctor who admitted them was a woman: Tsugawa, Y., et al., 'Comparison of Hospital Mortality and Readmission Rates for Medicare Patients Treated by Male vs Female Physicians,' *JAMA Intern Med*, 177:2 (2017), pp. 206–213.

197   Professor Jane Dacre concluded that medicine is 'richer' for diversity in its workforce in: Dacre, J., 'We need female doctors at all levels and in all specialties,' *BMJ* 344 (2012), 10.1136/bmj.e2325.

A group of researchers from Oxford University concluded medicine needs to establish career paths that enable both sexes to train and work part-time: Lachish, S., et al., 'Factors associated with less-than-full-time working in medical practice: results of surveys of five cohorts of UK doctors, 10 years after graduation,' *Hum Resour Health* 14:1 (2016), 10.1186/s12960-016-0162-3.

Professor Fiona Karet Frankl in: Karet Frankl,E. F., 'To be or not to be ... ' *Postgrad Med J* 92 (2016), p. 569–570.

Risky Business

202   Psychologist Kath Woolf's description of negative stereotypes in: Woolf, K., et al., 'Ethnic stereotypes and the underachievement of UK medical students from ethnic minorities: qualitative study,' *BMJ* 337 (2008), 10.1136/bmj.a1220.

205   Following the incident at Cardiff University, Dinesh Bhugra led an Independent Review Panel (2017). The report is available online at: https://www.cardiff.ac.uk/__data/assets/pdf_file/0011/551837/Prof-Dinesh-Bhugra-report-Final.pdf

John Dovidio's: Dovidio, J., 'The subtlety of racism,' *Train Dev J*, 47: 4 (1993), pp.50–57.

The 2017 BBC interview with Professor Robert Kelly, available online at: http://www.bbc.co.uk/news/world-asia-39244325.

206 Physicians discounted based on their skin colour, gender or both: Cooke, M., 'Implicit Bias in Academic Medicine,' *JAMA Intern Med*, 177:5 (2017), p.657.

207 Psychiatrist Damon Tweedy's account of being mistaken for a maintenance worker in: Tweedy, D., *Black Man in a White Coat* (New York: Picador, 2015).

Doctors' unconscious biases can impact the actual treatment decisions that they make: FitzGerald, C., and Hurst, S., 'Implicit bias in healthcare professionals: a systematic review,' *BMC Med Ethics*, 18:1 (2017), p.19.

A 2012 study reported that paediatricians with greater pro-white bias were more likely to agree with prescribing a narcotic medication for a white patient than an African-American patient: Sabin, J., and Greenwald, A., (2012). 'The Influence of Implicit Bias on Treatment Recommendations for 4 Common Pediatric Conditions: Pain, Urinary Tract Infection, Attention Deficit Hyperactivity Disorder, and Asthma,' *Am J Public Health*, 102:5 (2012), pp. 988–995.

209 Authors Steele and Aronson reported 'stereotype threat' in: Steele, C. M., and Aronson, J., 'Stereotype threat and the intellectual test performance of African-Americans,' *J Pers Soc Psychol* 69 (1995), pp. 797–811.

214 Damon Tweedy described his fears of his colleagues' views in: Tweedy, D., *Black Man in a White Coat* (New York: Picador, 2015).

215 BME doctors may be expected to be more involved in family crises than their white peers: Dickins, K., et al., 'The Minority Student Voice at One Medical School,' *Acad Med* 88:1 (2013), pp.73–79; Phoenix, A., and Husain, F., 'Parenting and ethnicity,' *Joseph Rowntree Foundation* (2007) available onlin

at: https://www.jrf.org.uk/sites/default/files/jrf/migrated/files/parenting-ethnicity.pdf.

216   Studies have shown that UK BME medical students feel less well prepared for the transition to work: Goldacre, M., et al., (2010). 'Views of junior doctors about whether their medical school prepared them well for work: questionnaire surveys,' *BMC Med Educ* 10:78 (2010). 10.1186/1472–6920-10–78.

A follow-up study on specialist psychotherapy services for doctors: Davies, R. S., et al., 'A sea change for sick doctors – how do doctors fare after presenting to a specialist psychotherapy service?' *JMH* 25:3 (2016), pp. 238–244.

218   Figures from (UK) HESA available online at: https://www.hesa.ac.uk/data-and-analysis/students.

Figures from the (US) National Center for Education Statistics available online at: https://nces.ed.gov/fastfacts/display.asp?id=98. Specific medical school statistics from the US available online at: http://www.aamcdiversityfactsandfigures2016.org/.

Afro-Caribbean students are poorly represented in UK medical training: McManus, I., 'Medical school applicants from ethnic minority groups: identifying if and when they are disadvantaged,' *BMJ* 310:6978 (1995), pp. 496–500.

220   Kath Woolf's comprehensive study on ethnic differentials: Woolf, K., et al., 'Ethnicity and academic performance in UK trained doctors and medical students: systematic review and meta-analysis,' *BMJ* 342 (2011), 10.1136/bmj.d901.

An accompanying editorial by Professor Aneez Esmail: Esmail, A., 'Ethnicity and academic performance in the UK,' *BMJ* 342 (2011), 10.1136/bmj.d709.

Sir Richard Doll's research: Doll, R., and Hill, A., 'The Mortality of Doctors in Relation to Their Smoking Habits,' *BMJ* 1 (1954), pp.1451–1455.

221 A 2016 study from the GMC found that being an international medical graduate significantly increases the risk of failure. The study is available online at: http://www.gmc-uk.org/How_do_doctors_progress_through_key_milestones_in_training.pdf_67018769.pdf.

222 Open access data from the AAMC on MCAT scores by race/ethnicity is available online at: https://www.aamc.org/download/321498/data/factstablea18.pdf.

Socio-economic data from the AAMC by race/ethnicity is available online at: http://www.aamcdiversityfactsandfigures2016.org/report-section/section-3/.

Performance data from USMLE is available online at: http://www.usmle.org/performance-data/default.aspx#2016_overview.

223 A 2012 study of students found that black and African-American students were significantly more likely to fail STEP1 than their white peers: Andriole, D., and Jeffe, D., 'A National Cohort Study of U.S. Medical School Students Who Initially Failed Step 1 of the United States Medical Licensing Examination,' *Acad Med* 87:4 (2012), pp. 529–536.

MCAT scores are related to STEP1 scores: Brenner, J. M., et al., 'Formative Assessment in an Integrated Curriculum: Identifying At-Risk students for poor performance on USMLE Step 1 Using NBME Custom Exam Questions,' AAMC, *Proceedings of the 56th Annual Research in Medical Education Sessions* (2017), S21-25.

Charles Prober's explanation on the use of STEP1 scores: Prober, C., et al., 'A Plea to Reassess the Role of United States Medical Licensing Examination Step 1 Scores in Residency Selection,' *Acad Med* 9:1 (2016), pp.12–15.

STEP1 scores can discriminate against African-American appli cants: Edmond, M., Deschenes, J., et al., 'Racial Bias in Usin

346

USMLE Step 1 Scores to Grant Internal Medicine Residency Interviews,' *Acad Med*, 76:12 (2001), pp. 1253–1256.

224 The 2015 GMC's commitment to ensuring fair training pathways, available online at: http://www.gmc-uk.org/education/29478.asp. The GMC commissioned literature review: Plymouth University Peninsula., 'Understanding differential attainment across medical training pathways: A rapid review of the literature,' GMC (2015) available online at: http://www.gmc-uk.org/about/research/28332.asp.

225 The second GMC commissioned study: Woolf, K., et al., (2016). 'Fair Training Pathways for All: Understanding Experiences of Progression,' GMC (2016) available online at: http://www.gmc-uk.org/2016_04_28_FairPathwaysFinalReport. pdf_66939685.pdf.

229 The American Medical Association's official apology to African-American physicians: Aluko, Y., 'American Medical Association Apologizes for Racism in Medicine,' *J Natl Med Assoc* 100:10 (2008), pp. 1246–1247.
Acceptance into the Alpha Omega Alpha Honor Society: Boatright, D., et al., 'Racial Disparities in Medical Student Membership in the Alpha Omega Alpha Honor Society,' *JAMA Intern Med*, 177:5 (2017), p.659.

230 An invited commentary on the need for tracking allegedly race-neutral systems and advancement from: Cooke, M., 'Implicit Bias in Academic Medicine,' *JAMA Intern Med*, 177:5 (2017), p.657.

233 In 2016 the GMC reported that over a quarter of all doctors gained their primary medical qualification outside of the UK or Europe. The report is available online at: http://www.gmc-uk.org/ SOMEP_2016_Full_Report_Lo_Res.pdf_68139324.pdf
'What happens in medical school is a wider reflection on society,' wrote Professor Aneez Esmail in: Esmail, A., 'Ethnicity and academic performance in the UK,' *BMJ*, 342 (2011), 10.1136/bmj.d709.

234 Global information from HEFCE on the differences in student outcomes available online at: http://www.hefce.ac.uk/pubs/rereports/Year/2015/diffout/.

Over a ten-year period, the University of Texas Medical Branch introduced significant reforms: Lieberman, S., et al., 'Comprehensive Changes in the Learning Environment: Subsequent Step 1 Scores of Academically At-Risk Students,' *Acad Med*, 83: (10 suppl) (2008), S49-52.

235 The Cooper Medical School of Rowan University matriculated its first class: Personal Communication. I was directed towards this new medical school by a colleague at the AAMC who is involved with increasing the diversity of applicants admitted to medical school. Further information about the institution available at: www.rowan.edu/coopermed.

236 A 2017 article entitled 'Breaking the Silence': Acosta, D., and Ackerman-Barger, K., 'Breaking the Silence: Time to Talk about race and racism,' Acad Med 92:3 (2017), pp. 285–288.

No Exit

255 A 2013 survey carried out by a group of epidemiologists at Oxford University concluded that UK doctors rarely give up a medical career within twenty-five years of graduation: Goldacre, M. L., and Lamber, T. W., 'Participation in medicine by graduates of medical schools in the United Kingdom up to 25 years post graduation: national cohort surveys,' *Acad Med* 88:5 (2013), pp. 699–709.

In the US the 2015 Graduation Questionnaire reported that only 0.2% of respondents did not intend to practice medicine. The 2015 report is available online at: https://www.aamc.org/download/440552/data/2015gqallschoolssummaryreport.pdf.

UK teacher recruitment and retention information available online at: https://www.teachers.org.uk/edufacts/teacher-recruitment-and-retention.

256 The *Guardian* 2015 article: Campbell, D., 'Almost half of junior doctors reject NHS career after foundation training' available online at: https://www.theguardian.com/society/2015/dec/04/almost-half-of-junior-doctors-left-nhs-after-foundation-training.

The *Wall Street Journal* 2014 article entitled 'Why doctors are sick of their profession,' available online at: http://www.wsj.com/articles/the-u-s-s-ailing-medical-system-a-doctors-perspective-1409325361.

The total NHS investment in each fully qualified hospital consultant is estimated to be over half a million pounds: 'How much does it cost to train a doctor in the United Kingdom?' BMA (2013) available online at: https://www.bma.org.uk//media/Files/ ... /pressbriefing_cost_of_training_doctors.docx.

UKFPO Annual Reports 2010 and 2011, and F2 Careers Destination surveys for each year 2012–2016 inclusive are all available on the UKFPO website: www.foundationprogramme.nhs.uk.

Figures of UK doctors who have permanently left the profession available online at: www.foundationprogramme.nhs.uk.

257 The results from the BMA EU Survey of Doctors working in the UK are available at: https://www.bma.org.uk/collective-voice/policy-and-research/education-training-and-workforce/eu-doctors-survey.

Doctors' self-reported intention to leave practice reported in: Rittenhouse, D. R., et al., 'No exit: an evaluation of measures of physician attrition,' *Health Serv Res* 39:5 (2004), pp. 1571–1588.

A 2004 study carried out by the British Medical Association found that the decision to leave medicine is often traumatic: Cooke, L., and Chitty, A., 'Why do doctors leave the profession?' BMA, *Health Policy and Economic Research Unit* (2004).

264 A survey of emergency physicians in the US found that 64% reported feelings of guilt or inadequacy after unsuccessful pediatric resuscitation: Ahrens, W. R., and Hart, R. G., 'Emergency physicians' experience with pediatric death,' *Am J Emerg Med* 15:7 (1997), pp. 642–3.

A study of over 600 anaesthetists: Gazoni, M. F., et al., 'The impact of perioperative catastrophes on anesthesiologists: results of a national survey,' *Anesth Analg* 114:3 (2012), pp. 596–603.

A study of the impact of perinatal death on obstetricians: Gold, J. K., et al., 'How physicians cope with stillbirth or neonatal death: A national survey of obstetricians,' *Obstet Gynecol* 112:1 (2008), pp. 29–34.

266 The BMA small scale study of fourteen doctors: Cooke, L., and Chitty, A., 'Why do doctors leave the profession?' BMA, Health Policy and Economic Research Unit (2004).

267 Michael Crichton described leaving medicine in his essay 'Quitting medicine' in: Crichton, M., *Travels* (New York: Vintage Books, 2004).

269 Helen Rose Fuchs Ebaugh study: Ebaugh Fuchs, R. H., *Becoming an Ex: The Process of Role Exit* (Chicago & London: University Of Chicago Press, 1988).

Natural Selection

276 University of Oxford statistics available online at: https://www.ox.ac.uk/about/facts-and-figures/admissions-statistics.

The Medical Schools Council 'Guiding Principles for the Admission of Medical Students,' (Revised, March 2010) available online at: https://www.medschools.ac.uk/media/1931/guiding-principles-for-the-admission-of-medical-students.pdf.

276 In the UK, four-year graduate entry programmes comprise 10% of admissions: Garrud, P. (2011). 'Who applies and who gets admitted to UK graduate entry medicine? – an analysis of UK admission statistics,' *BMC Med Educ* 11:71 (2011),10.1186/1472–6920-11–71.

Low attrition rate statistics in: Yates, J., 'When did they leave, and why? A retrospective case study of attrition on the Nottingham undergraduate medical course,' *BMC Med Educ* 12:43 (2012); Maher, B. M., et al., 'Medical School Attrition – beyond the statistics. A Ten-year study,' *BMC Med Educ* 13:13 (2013),10.1186/1472–6920-13–13.

The AAMC reported in 2010 that approximately 3% of medical students do not complete their degrees. The report is available online at: https://www.aamc.org/download/165418/data/aibvol9_no11.pdf.pdf

Most students accepted to medical school end up graduating. An alternative explanation is known in the trade as the 'failure to fail': Cleland, J., et al., 'It is me or is it them? Factors that influence the passing of underperforming students,' *Med Educ* 42:8 (2008), pp. 800–9.

277 Yates' analysis of five consecutive intakes at Nottingham University Medical School in: Yates, J., and James, D., 'Predicting the "strugglers": a case-study of students at Nottingham University Medical School,' *BMJ* 332:1009 (2006), 10.1136/bmj.38730.678310.63.

The 2010 GMC study of doctors who were disciplined for professional misconduct: Yates, J., and James, D., 'Risk factors at medical school for subsequent professional misconduct: multicenter retrospective case-control study,' *BMJ* 340 (2010), 10.1136/bmj.c2040. Studies from the US, on doctors who were disciplined for professional misconduct by the State Licensing Board: Papadakis, M., et al., 'Unprofessional behaviors in medical school is associated with subsequent disciplinary action by a state medical board,' *Acad*

Med 79:3 (2004), pp. 244–9; Papadakis, M., et al., 'Disciplinary action by medical boards and prior behavior in medical school,' *N Engl J Med* 353 (2005), pp. 2673–2682.

278 Only a tiny proportion of doctors in the UK and USA end up being disciplined by the relevant regulator: Figures for the UK are available online at: https://www.gmc-uk.org/DC9491_07___ Fitness_to_Practise_Annual_Statistics_Report_2015___Publis hed_Version.pdf_68148873.pdf.

Figures for the US are available online at: https://www.fsmb. org/Media/Default/PDF/FSMB/Publications/us_medical_ regulato ry_trends_actions.pdf.

Jennifer Cleland, a physician and educator at Aberdeen Medical School, has researched the 'failure to fail' within the medical school training: Cleland, J., et al., 'It is me or is it them? Factors that influence the passing of underperforming students,' *Med Educ* 42:8 (2008), pp. 800–9.

280 Cleland questions the approach to remediating underperforming students in: Cleland, J., et al., 'The remediation challenge: theoretical and methodological insights from a systematic review,' *Med Educ* 47:3 (2013), pp. 242–51.

282 In the US, MCAT scores have routinely been shown to predict results on the first set of national examinations (STEP1): Brenner, J. M., et al., 'Formative Assessment in an Integrated Curriculum: Identifying At-Risk students for poor performance on USMLE Step 1 Using NBME Custom Exam Questions,'AAMC 92.11S. *Proceedings of the 56ᵗʰ Annual Research in Medical Education Sessions* (2017), S21-25.

The ability of MCAT scores to predict later clinical performance as a doctor seems to be extremely weak: Sagull, A., et al., 'Does the MCAT predict medical school and PGY-1 performance?' *Mil Med* 180: 4 (2015), pp. 4–11.

282–3 Chris McManus et al., discuss the 'academic backbone' in: McManus, C., et al., 'The academic backbone: longitudinal continuities in educational achievement from secondary school and medical school to MCRP (UK) and the specialist register in UK medical students and doctors,' *BMC Med* 11:242 (2013), 10.1186/1741–7015-11–242.

284 A national survey of first year foundation doctors found that 31% attended a private school. For further information see the *'Selecting for Excellence'* report, available online at: https://www.medschools.ac.uk/media/1203/selecting-for-excellence-final-report.pdf

A similar social bias is seen in the US with approximately half of medical students coming from families with the top 20% of income. Figures available online at: https://www.aamc.org/download/102338/data/aibvol8no1.pdf.

Since 2001, King's College London has admitted students from low-achieving secondary schools onto the Extended Medical Degree Programme (EMDP): Garlick, P., 'Widening participation in medicine,' *BMJ* 336:1111 (2008), 10.1136/bmj.d918.

284 In an article for the *Psychologist*, McManus et al., caution against lowering medical school entry grades: Woolf, K., McManus, C., et al., 'The best choice?' the *Psychologist* 28:9 (2015), pp. 730–734.

285 A five-year study of over six thousand entrants to Medical School in the UK: Tiffin, A. P., et al., 'Predictive validity of the UKCAT for medical school undergraduate performance: a national prospective cohort study,' *BMC Med* 14:140 (2016), 10.1186/s12916-016-0682-7.

An evaluation and case study of the Biomedical Admissions Test: McManus, I. C., et al., 'Predictive validity of the Biomedical Admissions Test: An Evaluation and case study,' *Med Teach* 33:1 (2011), pp. 53–7.

286–7 In 2012 the medical profession was named and shamed in this review: 'Fair Access to Professional Careers: A progress report by the Independent Reviewer on social mobility and child poverty,' (2012) available online at: https://www.gov.uk/government/publications/fair-access-to-professional-careers-a-progress-report.

287 A Scottish study found that GPs from less affluent backgrounds were more likely to work in deprived communities: Dowell, J., et al., 'Widening access to medicine may improve general practitioner recruitment in deprived and rural communities: survey of GP origins and current place of work,' *BMC Med Educ* 15: 165 (2015), 10.1186/s12909-015-0445-8.

Students who study in a more diverse medical school end up having more positive attitudes towards patients from minority groups: Saha, S., et al., 'Student Body Racial and Ethnic Composition and Diversity-Related Outcomes in US Medical Schools,' *JAMA* 300: 10 (2008), pp. 1135–1145.

In 2014 the Medical Schools Council compiled a list of the key skills and attributes needed to study medicine, available online at: www.medschools.ac.uk.

Studies have asked patients what they look for in their doctor, for example: Wen, S. L., et al., 'What do people want from their health care? A qualitative study,' *J Participat Med* 7: e10 (2015).

289 Cleland led a major review identifying best practice in the selection of medical students: Cleland, J., et al., 'Research Report: Identifying best practice in the selection of medical students,' GMC (2013) available at https://www.gmc-uk.org/about/research/25036.asp.

Guidance from the Medical Schools Council shows that the majority of UK medical schools no longer score personal statements: 'Entry requirements for UK medical schools 2017 entry,' Medical Schools Council (2017) available online at https://www.medschools.ac.uk/media/2357/msc-entry-requirements-for-uk-medical-schools.pdf.

290 An exploratory study of which eleven-year olds would like to become a doctor: McManus, C., et al., 'Doctor, builder, soldier, lawyer, teacher, dancer, shopkeeper, vet: exploratory study of which eleven-year olds would like to become a doctor,' *BMC Psychol* 3:38 (2015), 10.1186/s40359-015-0094-z.

The impact of unconscious bias has been found to be a significant factor in interviews for other professions: Howard, J. R., *Everyday Bias: Identifying and Navigating Unconscious Judgements in Our Daily Lives* (Lanham: Rowman & Littlefield, 2014).

Icahn School of Medicine in New York are doing unconscious bias training for all interview panel members. (Personal communication with author).

A study in a medical school in the Midwest found that all members had significant unconscious bias for white people: Capers, Quinn IV; Clinchot, D., et al., 'Implicit Racial Bias in Medical School Admissions,' *Acad Med* 92:3 (2017), pp. 365–369.

293 In 2004, Professor Kevin Eva and his colleagues at McMaster University adopted the multiple mini interview format: Eva, W. K., et al., 'An admissions OSCE: the multiple mini-interview,' *Med Educ* 38:3 (2004), pp. 314–26.

296 In the UK, MMIs were piloted by Dundee Medical School: Dowell, J., et al., 'The multiple mini-interview in the UK context: 3 years of experience at Dundee,' *Med Teach* 34:4 (2012), pp. 297–304.

297 Kevin Eva followed up with the original MMI cohort in: Eva, W. K., et al., 'Association between a Medical School Admission Process Using the Multiple Mini-interview and National Licensing Examination Scores,' *JAMA* 308: 21 (2012), pp. 2233–2240.

In 2011, the great and the good in the world of medical education produced a consensus statement on medical school selection: Prideaux, D., et al., 'Assessment for selection for the health care professions and specialty training: consensus statement and recommendations from Ottawa 2010 Conference,' *Med Teach* 33.3 (2011), pp. 215–23.

298 Around the world, medical schools' desire to apply rigorous standards of evidence to their admissions processes: Dowell, J., et al., 'The multiple mini-interview in the UK context: 3 years of experience at Dundee,' *Med Teach* 34:4 (2012), pp. 297–304.

Chris McManus contributed to the global consensus statement on best practice in selection in: Prideaux, D., et al., 'Assessment for selection for the health care professions and specialty training: consensus statement and recommendations from Ottawa 2010 Conference,' *Med Teach* 33:3 (2011), pp. 215–23.

Donald Barr, writing in *The Lancet*: 'The art of medicine: Science as superstition: selecting medical students,' *The Lancet* 376 (2010), pp. 678–679.

299 Unprofessional behavior (such as lying) has been shown to increase the risk of subsequent action once the student has qualified: Papadakis, M. A., et al., 'Disciplinary action by medical bboards and prior behavior in medical school,' *N Engl J Med* 353: 25 (2005), pp. 2673–2682.

301 According to guidance from the GMC and the Medical Schools Council (2015), serious health issues will not jeopardize a career in medicine: 'Supporting Students with Mental Health Conditions' available online at: https://www.gmc-uk.org/Supporting_students_with_mental_health_conditions_0816.pdf_53047904.pdf.

302 Some medical schools advocate using a screening questionnaire: Powis, A. D., 'Selecting medical students: An unresolved challenge,' *Med Teach* 37:3 (2014), pp. 252–60.

Organisations that assess whether staff will cope with extremely demanding assignments have developed sophisticated questionnaires. (Personal communication regarding the work of *Interhealt*

Worldwide – an international charity that provided medical, psychological, occupational and travel health to staff working in international development. The charity was founded in 1989 and sadly closed in 2017 due to financial challenges).

Epilogue

308 The video of the liver transplant operation is available online at: https://www.theguardian.com/society/video/2016/feb/08/ living-donor-liver-transplant-from-son-to-father-video

310 The mantra of 'patient-centred care' from The National Institute for Clinical Excellence (NICE) outlines what patient-centred care involves, available online at: https://www.nice.org.uk/guidance/ cg161/chapter/patient-centred-care

311 Paediatrician and psychoanalyst Donald Winnicott in: Winncott, D., 'Further thoughts on babies as persons,' in Hardenberg, J., ed., *The child and the outside world: Studies in developing relationships* (London: Tavistock Publications Ltd, 1957 [original work published 1949]).

312 In a classic paper, Winnicott lists eighteen reasons why a mother may, at times, experience hateful feelings towards her baby: Winnicott, D., 'Hate in the Counter-Transference,' *Int J Psychoanal* 30 (1949), pp. 69–74.

315 One hundred and fifty years ago, the surgeon Joseph Lister published his findings on using antiseptics: Jackson, M., *The History of Medicine: A Beginner's Guide* (London: Oneworld, 2014).

316 'Resilience is always contextual' state the authors of a recent article in the *BMJ*: Balme, E., et al., 'Doctors need to be supported, not trained in resilience,' *BMJ* Careers (2015) available online at: http://careers.bmj.com/careers/advice/Doctors_need_to_be_ supported,_not_trained_in_resilience.

BRIEF GLOSSARY OF
UK MEDICAL TERMS

BMA	British Medical Association – the doctors' professional union
BMJ	*British Medical Journal*
EPM	Educational Performance Measure (used in Foundation Application)
F1	Foundation Year 1. 1st year of clinical practice after leaving medical school. Doctors are provisionally registered with the GMC at this point in their career
F2	Foundation Year 2. 2nd year of clinical practice after leaving medical school. Doctors are fully registered with the GMC at this point.
GMC	General Medical Council. National organization responsible for the licensing of doctors
IMG	International Medical Graduate
MSC	Medical Schools Council
SJT	Situational Judgement Test – a multiple-choice assessment of professional judgements
Trust Grade	Doctor delivering a clinical service, but not on a career progression ladder

UKFPO   United Kingdom Foundation Programme Office. The organization responsible for the management of the two-year foundation programme across the UK.

TRANSLATE → # TRAINING CHART

Simplified Map of Medical Training in the UK

Take UK Clinical Admissions Test (UCAT) or Biomedical Admissions Test (BMAT)

↓

MEDICAL SCHOOL
4 years: graduate entry programmes
5 years: standard undergraduate programme
6 years: standard undergraduate programme and intercalated degree

↓

Application to Foundation Programme

↓

FOUNDATION TRAINING
F1: Provisional registration with General Medical Council (GMC)
F2: Full registration with GMC

↓

SPECIALTY TRAINING 3-8 years	NON-TRAINING POSTS Delivering a clinical service but not progressing to complete training

↓

Certificate of Completion of Training (CCT)
Eligible to be on Specialist or GP Register

↓

Appointed hospital consultant or GP

↓

Continuing Professional Development (CPD) throughout career

FURTHER READING

Balint, Enid; Courtenay, Michael; Elder, Andrew; Hull, Sally and Julian, Paul. *The Doctor, the Patient and the Group*. London: Routledge, 1993

Ballatt, John & Campling, Penny. *Intelligent Kindness*. London: RCPsych Publications, 2011

Carel, Havi. *Illness*. London: Routledge, 2014

Cassell, Eric J. *The nature of Suffering and the Goals of Medicine*. Oxford: Oxford University Press, 1991

Cassell, Joan. *The Woman in the Surgeon's Body*. Cambridge, Mass: Harvard University Press, 1998

Charon, Rita. *Narrative Medicine*. Oxford: Oxford University Press, 2008

Gawande, Atul. *Complications*. London: Profile Books, 2002

Gawande, Atul. *Being Mortal*. London: Profile Books, 2015

Groopman, Jerome. *How Doctors Think*. Boston: Houghton Mifflin, 2008

Kalanithi, Paul. *When Breath becomes Air*. London: Bodley Head, 2016

Katz, Jay. *The silent World of Doctor and Patient*. Baltimore, MD: The Johns Hopkins University Press, 2002

Kleinman, Arthur. *The illness narratives*. New York: Basic Books, 1988

Main, Tom. *The Ailment and Other Psychoanalytic Essays*. London: Free Association Books, 1998

Marsh, Henry. *Do No Harm*. London: Weidenfeld & Nicholson, 2014

Maunder, Robert & Hunter, Jonathan. *Love, Fear and Health*. Toronto: University of Toronto Press, 2015

Montross, Christine. *Falling into the Fire*. London: Oneworld, 2014

Neighbor, Roger. *The Inner Physician*. London: Royal College of Physicians, 2016

Ofri, Danielle. *What Doctors Feel*. Boston: Beacon Press, 2013

Pringle, Rosemary. *Sex and Medicine*. Cambridge: Cambridge University Press, 2011

Ross, Howard J. *Everyday Bias*. Lanham, MD: Rowman & Littlefield, 2014

Sinclair, Simon. Making Doctors. Oxford: Berg, 1997

Sontag, Susan. *Illness as Metaphor*. London, Penguin Classics, 2002

Straker, Norman (Ed). *Facing Cancer and the Fear of Death*. Lanham, MD: Jason Aronson, 2013

Subotsky, Fiona; Bewley, Susan & Crowe, Michael. (Eds). *Abuse of the doctor-patient relationship*. London: RCPsych Publications, 2010

Tweedy, Damon. *Black Man in a White Coat*. New York: Picador, 2015

Vaillant, George E. *Adaptation to Life*. Cambridge, Mass: Harvard University Press, 1995

Watermeyer, Brian. *Towards a Contextual Psychology of Disabilism*. London: Routlege, 2013

ACKNOWLEDGEMENTS

The generosity with which the doctors in this book have allowed me to share their stories is astounding; my largest debt of gratitude goes to them. To protect their anonymity, I cannot acknowledge them by name, and even though each has given me permission to tell their story, I have also gone to great lengths to protect their identity. However I want each and every one of them to know how deeply grateful I am. I also want to acknowledge how many of these doctors were motivated to share their stories through altruism; in their emails back to me, after I had sent them what I had written, a number expressed satisfaction that their story might be used to benefit future generations of doctors. The following example is typical: 'Given my experience I am so grateful that mine and other trainee doctors' experiences are being highlighted and I really hope this will effect much needed changes in the system.' I hope so too.

I couldn't give a precise figure for the number of doctors I have supported in the two different roles described in this book – but it is definitely over six hundred. Whilst I have only told the stories of a small fraction of this total, all the other encounters, both consciously and unconsciously, have informed my understanding of the psychological demands of medical work. And although I owe a special debt of gratitude to those doctors who agreed to be included in the book, I also want to acknowledge how much I learnt in my first job, when I was tasked with observing doctors at work, and also in my second one, when doctors came to talk to me about the difficulties that they were experiencing in their medical careers.

Thankfully in both of these roles, I didn't work alone. I am inordinately grateful to Danë Goodsman who gave me my first job in medical education and from whom I learnt so much. It was Danë who came up with the radical idea that if you want to improve the quality of medical teaching it is far more effective to send trained faculty to observe doctors at work, than to extract these doctors from their hospital duties, plonk them in a classroom and subject them to lectures on 'top tips' of teaching. In this role, I also benefitted from the wisdom of Joan Reid, Pam Shaw and, until her untimely death, Kath Green. The ten years that I spent observing doctors at work laid the foundation for everything that came later.

In 2008 I jumped ship and moved to London Deanery, to set up the Careers Unit; many of the stories in this book are of doctors who sought support from that service. I am particularly grateful to Andrew Long, who was the senior clinician working alongside me to set up the Careers Unit and who has always been a great source of practical advice. My two administrators – Nicola Greaves and later Franco Henwood also played an important part; those who know me well would attest to the fact that administration has never been my forte. Philippa Shallard, former Manager of the North West Thames Foundation School based at Imperial College helped me with the chapter on transition from medical school. Camilla Kingdom and Suni Perera have also both been exceptionally generous with their support, encouraging me, answering my annoying questions and checking the clinical content of stories. Suni Perera, in addition, gave me the opportunity to co-facilitate two Balint groups – I found this work fascinating, have written a bit about it in the book and hope to do more of it, now that the book is finished. I would also like to mention the important role that my colleague Kath Sullivan played, particularly in the early stages of writing this book.

Beyond my immediate colleagues at the deanery, I have benefitted from the expertise of Clare Gerada and her team at the Practitioner Health Programme, as well as Julia Bland from DocHealth. I would also like to thank two colleagues from UCL Medical School: Anne Griffin who helped me with the section on dissection and Kath Woolf who read the chapter on racism in medicine; the latter rightly questioned my use of the term 'non-white'. 'Would you like to be referred to as non-male?' she asked.

In 2011 I was awarded a travelling fellowship by the Association for the Study of Medical Education, and went to work with psychologist Nicole Borges, a leading medical education researcher in the US. Nicole and I collaborated on an academic book chapter, and also co-facilitated a workshop at a conference organized by AAMC – the Association of American Medical Colleges. In addition to support from Nicole, contacts at AAMC such as George Richard and Sarah Conrad have been exceptionally generous with their time, and have helped me enormously with research into medical training in the US. Sarah Conrad also identified medical schools in the US with innovative approaches to widening diversity; in turn conversations with Marlene Ballejos and Robert Sapien at the School of Medicine, University of New Mexico and also with Jocelyn Mitchell-Williams at Cooper Medical School, Rowan University gave me inspiring examples of what medical schools can achieve, when there is a commitment to change from the top.

That old adage 'if you want something done, ask a busy person' has consistently been confirmed whilst writing this book. Many practitioners have been exceptionally generous in sharing their time and expertise; often it is those in the most senior positions, who responded first. In the UK I would like to acknowledge wonderful conversations with Susan Bewley, Aneez Esmail, Michael Farquhar and Jyoti Shah. I also approached Domhnall Macauley based in Northern Ireland, after I read his blog post entitled 'A young doctor's death'. In the course of that conversation I realized how angry I felt about the loss of life through suicide, in the early years of medical training. Domhnall encouraged me to hold onto the anger, rather than adopt a more neutral, academic tenor – a suggestion which I found particularly liberating.

But I didn't only benefit from contacts close to home – clinicians and researchers from across the globe were extraordinarily helpful. In the US, Howard Ross, an expert on implicit bias had a lengthy conversation with me and then pointed me in the direction of Pamela Abner, a diversity specialist at Mount Sinai Health System in New York City. Johanna Shapiro, a psychologist researching empathy was generous with her time, and helped me write the chapter on trauma and the erosion of empathy. Brian Watermeyer, a psychologist based at the University of Cape Town wrote an astonishing book on disability; a subsequent conversation with him helped with the 'Role Reversal' chapter.

In addition to learning from senior practitioners, a number of junior doctors have also read and commented on different chapters. In the UK I am particularly grateful for the input of Senem Sahin, Jemma Saville and Meenakshi Verma, whilst in the US, Anna Kuan-Celarier was wonderfully patient at answering my email queries. Rebecka Fleetwood-Smith, a psychology PhD student who will surely go far, helped with literature searches, and also was fantastically efficient in compiling the final version of the 'Notes'.

As a psychologist, I've depended on regular monthly supervision from an experienced colleague. I would like to acknowledge how much I've learnt over the years from Rob Nathan, who supervised my work with many of the doctors described in this book. More recently I have enormously enjoyed being supervised by Mary Burd who combines a deep psychodynamic understanding with considerable experience of supporting junior doctors. I also want to mention how much I learnt from Pam Howard and Lawrence Suss; the two best teachers I have ever had, and without whose input, I would not have been able to write about anyone's inner life.

In addition to my professional work in medical education, the experience of being a patient has also informed my understanding of what it takes to be a good doctor. GPs don't always get a good press but the doctors at Keats Group Practice are excellent and I am particularly grateful to Drs Lucia Grun and Eunice Laleye for their sensitive way in which they have looked after my physical and mental health over the past twenty-five years. Growing up with an autistic sibling posed its own set of challenges, and the input of Professor Sir Michael Rutter and his colleagues at the Maudsley Hospital, again over very many years, made a huge difference to all of our family. More recently I have benefited from Howard Cooper's exceptional skills as a psychotherapist. The capacity to understand somebody else's inner life – crucial for writing a book of this kind – critically depends upon the capacity to appreciate one's own; his sustained support, in so many ways, helped me complete this book.

Many friends also played a part. Claire Elliott and Sarah Thurlbeck, answered many medical questions; when I felt that I couldn't bother colleagues any more, these two dear friends stepped into the breech. Suzanne Franks played a crucial role right at the beginning, and without her support, I would have abandoned the project. Alison Donaldson was also incredibly helpful in the early stages of writing. Nat Janz has a rare combination of psychological and publishing expertise, and many writing blocks were dissolved on walks across the heath. Sometimes we had the good fortune to be joined by Katy Steward, who brought a nuanced understanding of organisational issues in healthcare to the discussion. Both Nat and Mark Ellingham also helped with decisions about the cover. When writing the epilogue the experience of Ruth and Noam Tamir came to mind and I would like to acknowledge my gratitude to both of them for allowing me to share their family's experience of live donor liver transplantation.

This book would never have happened without a chance conversation with the literary agent, Patrick Walsh. 'Why don't you write a book?' Patrick asked me as we were both leaving BMA House, following the Annual BMA Book Awards. 'Actually I've started on a proposal,' I replied as we headed off in different directions. I thought no more about this until a couple of days later when Patrick emailed and asked me to send him what I had written. I am particularly grateful for the way in which Patrick pushed me to improve the initial proposal; with the benefit of his expertise, it was sharpened up beyond recognition. Then, to my great delight, Tom Avery at William Heinemann bought the book. I couldn't have asked for a better editor as Tom combines kindness and positivity with exceptional editorial skills. The difference between the first and final drafts of this book is remarkable and almost entirely down to Tom's insightful editorial input. Kate McQuaid, the Publicity Director at William Heinemann has been fantastic to work with, and I would also like to acknowledge the patience of the design team who had to produce numerous different cover options before we ended up with one that everyone was happy with.

And finally, my family – Michael, Jonathan, Miriam and Andrew Franklin. Some family members were early adopters of the idea that I might write this book, whilst others took far longer to come on board. Irrespective of their initial response, in the end everyone helped, be it through the provision of 24/7 technical support, late-night conversations around the kitchen table on how the racial context is different in the UK and the US, sourcing obscure references, offering perceptive feedback on title options, encouraging me when it all felt too difficult and sharing their editorial expertise. Even my two grandchildren (who were both born during the course of writing the book) played a part. Admittedly neither of them had much to say about the inner lives of doctors, but grandchildren proved to be the perfect antidote to the loneliness of writing. And entirely serendipitously, with one born in the UK and the other in the US, their arrivals gave me a more personal sense of how the culture of medicine differs between the two countries. I am inordinately grateful for the love and support that each family member has given me – this book is for them.